Patents: a basic guide
to patenting in biotechnology

R. S. CRESPI
British Technology Group

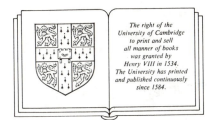

*The right of the
University of Cambridge
to print and sell
all manner of books
was granted by
Henry VIII in 1534.
The University has printed
and published continuously
since 1584.*

CAMBRIDGE UNIVERSITY PRESS

Cambridge

New York   New Rochelle

Melbourne   Sydney

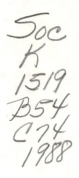

Published by the Press Syndicate of the University of Cambridge
The Pitt Building, Trumpington Street, Cambridge CB2 1RP
32 East 57th Street, New York, NY 10022, USA
10 Stamford Road, Oakleigh, Melbourne 3166, Australia

First published 1988

Printed in Great Britain at the University Press, Cambridge

British Library cataloguing in publication data

Crespi, R.S. (R. Stephen)
Patents: a basic guide to patenting in
biotechnology. – (Cambridge studies in
biotechnology; 6).
1. Biotechnology. Patents. Legal aspect
I. Title
342.64'86

Library of Congress cataloguing in publication data

Crespi, R. S.
Patents: a basic guide to patenting in biotechnology/R.S. Crespi.
p.   cm. – (Cambridge studies in biotechnology: 6)
Includes index.
ISBN 0 521 32954 X
1. Biotechnology – Patents.   I. Title.   II. Series.
K1519.B54C74 1988 346.04'86 – dc19 [342.6486]

ISBN 0 521 32954 X

Contents

Preface

Basic outlines of patent law for research workers in chemistry and the biological sciences are available in textbooks and the scientific journals. These contributions have been more frequent in recent years with the increasing emphasis on biotechnology as an opportunity for innovation and new industrial growth. Nevertheless the demand for a simplified presentation on patents is still heard and is understandable. The research worker in biotechnology, being already hard pressed to keep up with his own rapidly developing subject, is in need of relatively easy access to answers to the many questions that arise if and when he starts to think at all seriously about patents. This introduction to patenting in biotechnology attempts to provide this information in a convenient form and through dialogue. Thus a question and answer presentation is used to convey a legal understanding sufficient for the needs of the research worker or other non-lawyer working in an area of basic or applied research which may conceivably lead to innovation in industrial processes and products.

Patent law exists to serve technology, not to be its master, and its justification rests entirely on that foundation. Recent criticism of the patent system as 'arcane' can be answered in part by removing obscurities which may inhibit close encounter with its ideas and practices. Some who are not particularly well informed on the subject can still hold firm views about what ought or ought not to be allowed in the way of patent protection, as the dialogues presented here will show. In addition to answering questions some formal explanations of various facets of patent law are also given interspersed with examples and specific cases by way of illustration. The object being to explain the ideas current in patent law and practice, the text has not been burdened with detailed references to statutes and cases such as a patent lawyer would want to see. The interested reader who wishes to go further into the sources will be able to do so by consulting the further reading list given at the end of this book.

R.S.C.
October 1987

1 Awareness of intellectual property

For many scientists the subject of patents and other forms of intellectual property is thought to be mysterious, unnecessarily complex, and best avoided. This attitude is widespread and not peculiar to scientific workers in biotechnology.

The concepts and procedures of patent law are commonly dismissed as an esoteric activity indulged in only by those who enjoy hair-splitting distinctions and tortuous argument. Although this judgement is distorted, there is no doubt that the law covering the patenting of inventions has its share of 'dry dust' and complex rules and regulations. Biotechnology, however, has brought the patent law to life in more senses than one. The idea of patenting 'life' has had a peculiar fascination for the philosophically-minded, and it is not without interest also for the ordinary person who sees it as part of the intervention of science in the control of life processes. For lawyers and legislators biotechnology inventions have raised questions to which traditional patent law does not offer easy solutions, and these have stimulated a movement towards a re-examination of the fundamentals of patent law and their application to innovation in microbiology.

The current concern over the general lack of awareness of intellectual property is based on the belief that this subject ought to be more in the minds of those upon whom we depend for new technology. While new technology is being nursed into infancy and beyond it is important for those who invest in this risky process to have available the protection of patents and other forms of intellectual property which will ensure that once a market is established for a new product or process it will not be pirated by those who have not laboured to bring it to birth.

The research worker in science and technology does not easily acquire a working knowledge of the basic do's and don'ts of patent law and often learns of these by painful experience. In the crowded curricula of universities and other institutes of higher education, it is impossible to do more than make bare mention of ways and means of handling discoveries which the postgraduate worker may make in the course of a subsequent research career. In industry the research worker will, sooner or later, have to give some thought to the question of patents or other forms of legal protection. Even here, however, the extent of awareness in industry is patchy and unless the company has a substantial Research

1

and Development investment justifying its own internal patent officer or patent department it may be difficult for the individual research worker to find out what he needs to know. For those in academic institutions the problem is a different one. Although academics might claim that their informational needs on this topic are not completely met there are now more opportunities than ever of access to basic information and practical help, given the appropriate degree of motivation on the part of the research worker. In biotechnology there has been a demand for patent specialists to provide articles in scientific journals, to contribute papers to the many seminars and conferences held on biotechnology, and generally to assume the role of communicators in this respect to a much greater extent than in the past and more so than for any other technology.

In reality the scientists need grasp little more than a few basic ideas of patent law. What is more important is to know when to seek professional advice. The researcher ought in the first place to have sufficient intuition to identify in the results emerging from research the elements of originality and practical utility which may be the basis of a new process or product of some economic interest. However so many research workers have been focussed throughout their scientific training upon goals and ideals which are more academic than practical in nature that it is common for them not to see the commercial potential of their work until it has been pointed out to them after publication. A major problem to be addressed, therefore, is how to recognise a patentable invention when one has turned up. This will not be achieved in a single chapter and indeed is one of the goals of this book as a whole.

In the following chapters no previous knowledge of this subject will be assumed and nothing more will be expected than a modest level of curiosity about its bare essentials. Although the subject will be approached from the point of view of those who are specialising or are already specialist in biotechnology it will be necessary to begin with basic features which are common to inventions in all technologies. Inevitably in an elementary treatment of a branch of law that can undeniably become complex in its application it is necessary to make approximate statements. This is especially so when dealing with the subject internationally as most statements about patent law are qualified by differences among the various national laws. Over much of the world, however, there is a common core of ideas and practices which if grasped is sufficient for the purposes of the research worker as inventor. Inventors may safely leave the more intricate points of difference to the professional patent lawyer whose services will usually be found indispensable in practice especially if international protection is required. Much of this presentation is in dialogue form based on the typical questions which occur to research groups working in universities or in industry and which any speaker on this subject can expect to receive from the younger audiences.

The patent system may be remote and arcane but only to those who will not approach it. The purpose of this work is to entice the newcomer into making contact with a subject which is too important to be left to patent lawyers alone. Before discussing the questions that most commonly concern research workers certain basic facts about the system as a whole should be seen in outline summary form:

The nature of patents

A patent is a property right granted by State Authority which excludes others from the use or benefit of the patented invention without the consent of the patentee. A patent does not confer a positive right to use an invention because freedom of use may be dependent on prior rights. For example a patent for an improvement on a basic product or process will often be subject to a prior patent for the basic product or process.

The patent application

To obtain a patent an application must be filed with the relevant national authority (Patent Office) and will be examined for compliance with legal requirements. After a process of negotiation between the applicant and the Patent Office Examiner the application will be accepted or rejected. This examination is principally concerned with the written specification of the invention which must be filed with the application and which must define the scope of the protection sought. Separate patent applications are usually necessary in each country where protection is required but a single application in the European Patent Office can cover a number of European countries up to the point at which rights are granted.

Patentability

Among the principal legal requirements for patentability there are four basic requirements, three of which the invention itself must fulfil, namely, it must have (1) novelty, (2) inventiveness and (3) practical utility or industrial applicability while the other (4) concerns the specification; this must be adequate in content to enable those of ordinary skill and experience in the field to follow the directions and obtain the promised results. The invention is defined in the 'claims' which form part of the specification. Common forms of claim are directed to an *apparatus* or *device*, a *process* or *product* of manufacture, a *composition*, and a *method* of treatment, testing or use.

Official examination

The Patent Office will carry out a search of previously published documents including the scientific and patent literature to determine the relevant 'prior art'. Following this the application will be examined in the light of the search results. This usually involves argument about the specification, especially the scope of the claims, and may take considerable time to settle.

Opposition or re-examination

Even after acceptance by the Patent Office a patent application or patent can in most countries be opposed by third parties who may raise objections and prior art similar to or additional to those already overcome by the applicant. This is usually termed Opposition and involves argument between the applicant/patentee and Opponent who have equal status as contending parties. US patent law does not provide for opposition in this sense but allows a third party to request official Re-examination of the patent in the light of prior art.

Duration of a patent

The term of a patent differs from country to country. In most European countries the term is 20 years from the *application* date. In the USA and Canada a patent lasts 17 years from *grant*. The payment of annual renewal fees is required in most countries to avoid lapsing of the protection.

The adversarial nature of the patenting process is the main reason for the time and cost entailed in obtaining results. The rights of inventors to seek and acquire a reasonable measure of protection for their contributions to technology have to be balanced against the also important rights of others to engage in industry and commerce without unfair restrictions on their technological freedom. Some tension is therefore inevitable. The approach taken in this book is unashamedly pro-inventor and pro-patent. A patent confers a monopoly without establishing itself a situation which can be described as Monopoly. That is, a patent provides an exclusive right to the use and enjoyment of a *particular* invention. It does not monopolise anything more than the specific invention, does not preclude alternative and different methods of solving the same problem, and is not anti-competitive but on the contrary stimulates competition and the search for ways to 'design around' the patent. It is therefore a reasonable right to allow to those who invent and thereby enrich the state of the art.

2   Introducing the patent system

At the outset of this enquiry the questions that arise for the research worker relate to the nature of patents and their relevance to science and technology. How useful patents can be and whether they are worth the time, expense, and trouble to obtain are questions that will follow closely upon the previous answers. If research workers conclude that the patent system expects too much from them they have two main alternatives. Either they may publish their work and therefore make it unpatentable for themselves and others or they may keep it secret and try to derive some benefit from the know-how. Whether these alternatives are open to the research worker will depend on the circumstances. It is hoped that the patent system will be given a fair trial. However, complete conviction on the questions that follow will not be achieved by discussion alone and can only come with experience of the actual handling or mishandling of inventions in real life.

1   Why should I take an interest in the subject of patents?

If you are working in pure or applied research either in industry or in an academic institution you may discover something which is not only of scientific interest but also solves an existing technological problem or makes some other contribution to new technology. Your findings may therefore have application to areas of practical utility and may be of significant economic value. Patents may be a way of realising this value in a form which could be of considerable advantage to yourself or your employer.

2   What exactly is a patent?

A patent is a form of property created by law and granted by appropriate authority. It gives to its owner a right of action against unauthorised use of the invention defined in it. It is one species of the general category of legal rights known as 'industrial property' or 'intellectual property' and is the type of right most appropriate for technological innovation.

5

3   **What does a patent look like?**

A patent is a document which usually consists of a cover page of a formal
kind attached to a specification of the invention. The cover page
announces or certifies that a patent has been granted and carries the
official seal or stamp of the Industrial Property Office. Examples of
such formal papers included in British, European and United States
patents are given below (Fig. 2.1–2.7).

4   **How does one obtain access to patent disclosures?**

Patents are published by the Government printer or equivalent in major
industrial countries. Copies can be ordered from the Sale Branch of the
Industrial Property Office by quoting the patent number or published
application number and upon payment of the appropriate fee which is
usually modest.

5   **Of what use is a patent?**

Mere possession of a patent is of relatively little use in itself. It is a
deterrent to others but this is only useful if you yourself are making
practical use of the invention and deriving some benefit from it.
Deterrence is a negative concept. A more positive approach is by active
exploitation of the invention in some way such as by licensing its use to
others. Where the invention is evidently of great value the world will
beat a path to your door. Usually, however, you will have to work to
persuade others to take up the idea and develop it to the point of
commercial application.

6   **How do patents relate to the practical application of research?**

We are postulating that the research has given rise to a new process or a
new product or a new type of device or apparatus or any other of the
recognised categories of patentable invention. The invention will have
to be adequately described and defined in the patent so that the rights
of the inventor or other owner of the patent are made clear with respect
to third parties. Any use which third parties wish to make of the defined
invention, especially where this is commercial use, will require the
consent of the patentee. Patents and other forms of industrial or
intellectual property provide legal mechanisms for the recognition of
the inventive rights of the research worker and also for the exploitation
of those rights such as by licensing and other forms of technology
transfer.

CERTIFICATE OF GRANT OF UNITED KINGDOM PATENT

In accordance with Section 24(2) of the Patents Act, 1977, it is hereby certified that a patent having the specification No 2160540 has been granted to National Research Development Corporation (United Kingdom) in respect of an invention disclosed in an application for that patent having a date of filing of 17 June 1985 being an invention for "Support material for immobilisation of ligands".

Dated this Twelfth day of August 1987

P. J. COOPER
Comptroller-General of Patents
Designs and Trade Marks

THE ATTENTION OF THE PROPRIETOR IS DRAWN TO THE IMPORTANT NOTES OVERLEAF

National Research Development Corporation
C/o R K Percy
Patents Department
101 Newington Causeway
London
SE1 6BU

053394

A

Fig. 2.1. Reproduced by kind permission of the Controller, H.M. Stationery Office.

IMPORTANT NOTES FOR PROPRIETORS OF UNITED KINGDOM PATENTS

1. **DURATION OF PATENT & PAYMENT OF RENEWAL FEES**

    (i)   A patent takes effect on the date shown at the foot of the certificate overleaf. Subject to the payment of renewal fees, it can be kept in force until the end of a period of 20 years from the date of filing the application for a patent.

    (ii)   To maintain the patent in force, it is necessary for the proprietor or someone on his behalf to pay a prescribed annual renewal fee. Payment may be made not more than three months before the expiration of the fourth or relevant succeeding year from the date of filing the application for a patent and should be accompanied by Patents Form 12/77.

    (iii) **The proprietor is responsible for ensuring that effective renewal arrangements are set up and maintained and that fees are paid on time.** He should not await any communication from the Patent Office before paying the fee; an official reminder sent to the last recorded address for service within six weeks **after** the anniversary of the date of the patent is intended to alert the proprietor to possible failure of his renewal arrangements.

    (iv)   If the form with the fee is not lodged in the Patent Office on or before the anniversary date of the patent, the fee cannot be accepted unless application for an extension of time to a maximum of 6 months is made and paid for on Patents Form 13/77. Thereafter if no renewal fee is received and no extension of time is requested, the patent will cease. No reduction of extension fees is made in the case of a patent endorsed "Licences of Right". When paying a renewal or extension fee it is advisable first to check the current scale of charges as these may change from time to time.

2. **PROCEDURE FOR PAYMENT OF FEES**

    Patents fees are payable direct to the Patent Office by means of cash, money order, postal order, banker's draft or cheque. (Adhesive stamps will not be accepted in payment of fees). The prescribed fee must be submitted together with the appropriate completed Patents Form; in addition each form or batch of forms should be accompanied by a fee sheet (FS. 1) showing details of the form(s) and the amount(s) of the fee(s). Cheques, money orders, etc., should be made payable to "The Comptroller-General, Patent Office", and crossed. Patents Forms, together with the fees and fee sheet (FS. 1) may be delivered to the Patent Office in London either by hand or post; those sent by post should be addressed to "The Cashier, The Patent Office, State House, 66-71 High Holborn, London WC1R 4TP".

    Blank Patents Forms and fee sheets (FS. 1) can be obtained from the Clerk of Stationery, The Patent Office, 25 Southampton Buildings, London WC2A 1AY".

3. **REGISTRATION OF OWNERSHIP AS EVIDENCE OF ENTITLEMENT**

    Any person who claims to have acquired the property in a patent by virtue of any transaction, instrument or event shall be entitled as against any other person who claims to have acquired that property by virtue of an earlier transaction, if application is made to the comptroller for registration in the register of patents (see Sections 32 and 33 of the Patents Act 1977). Particulars as to the manner of making such application may be obtained from the Patent Office.

Fig. 2.2. Reproduced by kind permission of the Controller, H.M. Stationery Office.

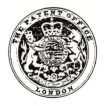

(12) **UK Patent** (19) **GB** (11) **2 160 540** (13) **B**

(54) Title of invention

Support material for immobilisation of ligands

(51) INT CL⁴; **C07G 7/00**

(21) Application No
8515265

(22) Date of filing
17 Jun 1985

(30) Priority data

(31) **8415666**

(32) **20 Jun 1984**

(33) **United Kingdom (GB)**

(43) Application published
24 Dec 1985

(45) Patent published
12 Aug 1987

(52) Domestic classification (Edition I)
C3U 2C7 4CX 4L
C3H 203 220 242 H1
U1S 1332 1614 C3H C3U

(56) Documents cited
None

(58) Field of search
C3U
C3H

(73) Proprietor
National Research Development Corporation

(Incorporated in United Kingdom),

101 Newington Causeway London SE1 6BU

(72) Inventors
Stephen Berezenko
Robert James Sturgeon

(74) Agent and/or
Address for Service
R. K. Percy,
Patents Department
National Research Development Corporation
101 Newington Causeway London SE1 6BU

LONDON THE PATENT OFFICE

GB 2 160 540 B

Fig. 2.3. Reproduced by kind permission of the Controller, H.M. Stationery Office.

Europäisches
Patentamt

European Patent
Office

Office européen
des brevets

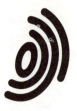

URKUNDE

Es wird hiermit bescheinigt, daß
für die in der beigefügten Patentschrift beschriebene Erfindung ein
europäisches Patent für die in der
Patentschrift bezeichneten Ver-
tragsstaaten erteilt worden ist.

CERTIFICATE

It is hereby certified that a
European patent has been granted
in respect of the invention
described in the annexed patent
specification for the Contracting
States designated in the specification.

CERTIFICAT

Il est certifié qu'un brevet
européen a été délivré pour
l'invention décrite dans le fascicule
de brevet ci-joint, pour les Etats
contractants désignés dans le
fascicule de brevet.

Europäisches Patent Nr.:
European patent No.:
Brevet européen n^o:

0123532

Patentinhaber:
Proprietor of the patent:
Titulaire du brevet:

NATIONAL RESEARCH DEVELOPMENT CORPORATION
101 Newington Causeway
London SE1 6BU/GB

F. KLEIN

München, den
Munich,
Fait à Munich, le

22.10.86

Generaldirektion 2 – Formalprüfungsstelle
Directorate-General 2 – Formalities Section
Direction générale 2 – Section des formalités

EPA/EPO/OEB Form 2031 03.83

Fig. 2.4.

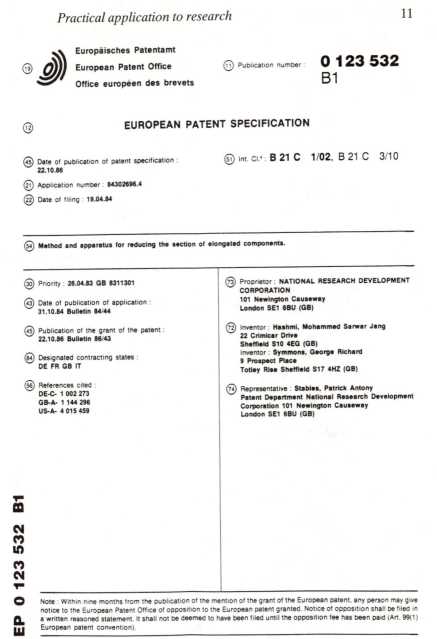

(19) Europäisches Patentamt
European Patent Office
Office européen des brevets

(11) Publication number : **0 123 532 B1**

(12) **EUROPEAN PATENT SPECIFICATION**

(45) Date of publication of patent specification :
22.10.86

(51) Int. Cl.⁴ : **B 21 C 1/02**, B 21 C 3/10

(21) Application number : 84302696.4

(22) Date of filing : 19.04.84

(54) Method and apparatus for reducing the section of elongated components.

(30) Priority : 26.04.83 GB 8311301

(43) Date of publication of application :
31.10.84 Bulletin 84/44

(45) Publication of the grant of the patent :
22.10.86 Bulletin 86/43

(84) Designated contracting states :
DE FR GB IT

(56) References cited :
DE-C- 1 002 273
GB-A- 1 144 296
US-A- 4 015 459

(73) Proprietor : NATIONAL RESEARCH DEVELOPMENT
CORPORATION
101 Newington Causeway
London SE1 6BU (GB)

(72) Inventor : Hashmi, Mohammed Sarwar Jang
22 Crimicar Drive
Sheffield S10 4EG (GB)
Inventor : Symmons, George Richard
9 Prospect Place
Totley Rise Sheffield S17 4HZ (GB)

(74) Representative : Stables, Patrick Antony
Patent Department National Research Development
Corporation 101 Newington Causeway
London SE1 6BU (GB)

EP 0 123 532 B1

Jouve, 18. rue St-Denis, 75001 Paris, France

Fig. 2.5.

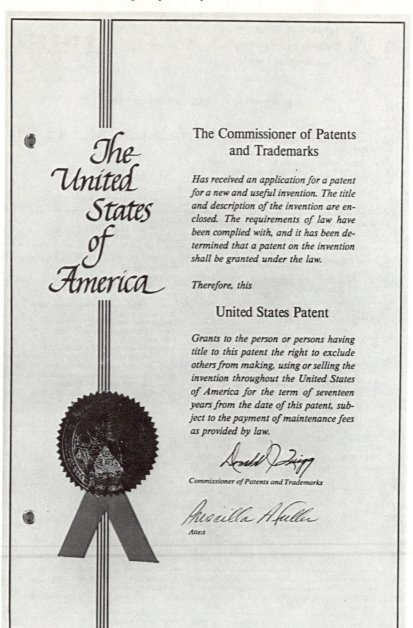

The Commissioner of Patents
and Trademarks

*Has received an application for a patent
for a new and useful invention. The title
and description of the invention are en-
closed. The requirements of law have
been complied with, and it has been determined that a patent on the invention
shall be granted under the law.*

Therefore, this

United States Patent

*Grants to the person or persons having
title to this patent the right to exclude
others from making, using or selling the
invention throughout the United States
of America for the term of seventeen
years from the date of this patent, subject to the payment of maintenance fees
as provided by law.*

Commissioner of Patents and Trademarks

Attest

Fig. 2.6.

United States Patent [19]

Spillman

[11] **Patent Number:** **4,660,762**

[45] **Date of Patent:** **Apr. 28, 1987**

[54] **METHOD AND APPARATUS FOR SPRAYING A TARGET SURFACE**

[75] Inventor: **John J. Spillman,** Bedford, England

[73] Assignee: **National Research Development Corporation,** London, England

[21] Appl. No.: **758,090**

[22] Filed: **Jul. 23, 1985**

[30] **Foreign Application Priority Data**

Jul. 23, 1984 [GB] United Kingdom 8418722

[51] Int. Cl.⁴ **B05B 15/04**
[52] U.S. Cl. **239/1;** 47/1.7; 239/172; 239/288; 244/136
[58] **Field of Search** 239/171, 172, 288–288.5, 239/1; 47/1.5, 1.7; 244/136

[56] **References Cited**

U.S. PATENT DOCUMENTS

3,512,714   5/1970   Phelps et al. .... 239/172 X
3,933,309   1/1976   Odegaard 239/171

FOREIGN PATENT DOCUMENTS

1513711   6/1978   United Kingdom .
2103251   2/1983   United Kingdom .

Primary Examiner—Andres Kashnikow
Attorney, Agent, or Firm—Cushman, Darby & Cushman

[57]   **ABSTRACT**

Method and apparatus for spraying a target surface, especially a penetrable surface like the canopy of a standing crop. The spray nozzles, mounted on a suitable vehicle, are moved over the surface and an arcuate shield, with its concave side facing towards the target, is mounted close to each nozzle on the side of that nozzle remote from the target. The effect of the movement of the shield upon the air lying between it and the target surface is to induce in that air a component of movement towards the surface, so improving the incidence upon the surface of the spray from the associated nozzle. The air movement may also tend to deflect the canopy, so helping to expose regions of the crop beyond the canopy. Such exposure can be promoted still further by mechanical deflectors. The arcuate shields may be of aerofoil section and the specification describes modified designs in which a shield comprises a series of elements with gaps between them, the envelope of all the elements having an aerofoil outline.

8 Claims, 7 Drawing Figures

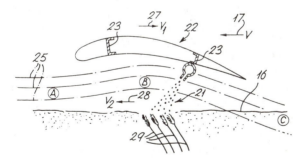

Fig. 2.7.

7   **Do patents stifle research? Is it not better to have free and open exchange of information and technology?**

A patent cannot stifle research because it does not prevent research as such. One can utilise the information in a patent so long as this is done in the context of research into the invention. This will be explained later when the question of infringement of the patentee's rights is considered.

Whether patents and other types of industrial property are beneficial overall is a part philosophical part pragmatic question. Philosophically

speaking it is difficult to see why a free-for-all should prevail in this area
when other forms of creativity are recognised as justifying a benefit to
their authors. Plagiarism is rightly regarded as undesirable. The patent
system provides an opportunity for inventors to benefit in return from
their contribution to technology. From the pragmatic angle a free-for-all
would only work if everyone played according to the same rules. There
is scant hope of achieving agreement on this. The test of the open system
would be whether it motivated research and investment in research
more than a system of proprietary rights is believed to do. This poses a
major burden of proof for the free-for-all philosopher. In adjudicating
on an antibiotic patent in 1971 the British House of Lords made the
following statement:

> 'Since the orginal discovery of the therapeutic uses of antibiotics
> and of the methods of aerobic fermentation by which they can
> be produced from micro-organisms to be found in nature,
> further advances in this field of medicine have been achieved
> by searching for and finding hitherto unidentified strains of
> micro-organisms existing in the natural state from which useful
> new antibiotics can be prepared by what is now a well-known
> standard process. The task of finding such a strain of micro-
> organisms calls for the exercise of technical proficiency and is
> laborious and very costly, for the odds against success are large.
> It is not easy to see what inventive step, as distinct from the
> mere exercise of proficiency and practice is involved in this kind
> of research, but the result of success in it is a new product useful
> to humanity which does not exist in nature. If such research is
> to be encouraged in a competitive society, the monetary rewards
> of success must be assured to those who undertake the expense;
> and the means of doing so in this and in most other countries
> with comparable social systems is by according to the successful
> discoverer of the new product the controlled and limited
> monopoly granted for inventions under the national patent
> laws.'

8   But does the patent system work effectively and really provide the motivation for innovation?

If it were not effective it would not survive on anything like its present
scale and its use would certainly not be on the increase. The results it
gives can be patchy and some inventors can be disappointed. There is
simply no uniform predictable pattern here and unless you travel the
road you will not know whether the journey is worthwhile. Although
certain stereotypes exist (one semi-synthetic penicillin patent can look
much like another) most patent agents will say that each case is different

and has to contend with its own prior art and inherent technical difficulties and other circumstances. Perhaps the real wisdom lies in trying to assess whether the system will deliver valuable results in your case or whether some other method of exploitation is more appropriate. A thorough knowledge of prior work and literature is essential to this assessment, as will appear later.

As to motivation it is widely known that the pharmaceutical industry will not undertake the costly development of new drugs without the prospect of a secure patent position which will extend for a significant period beyond the development phase and into the marketing phase. On the whole the patent system seems to work much better for the chemical and pharmaceutical industries than it does for engineers. It lends itself more to the grant of significant protection of enduring importance for key compounds or key intermediates. In engineering the ability to 'design around' a patent is less exceptional. The attitudes of the chemists and engineers themselves are also easily distinguishable.

9   **It sounds rather complicated nevertheless. Why cannot I simply concentrate on my research and let the patenting be done by an interested company or some other body?**

If you are an industrial worker you will find that some other member of company staff will take over much of the burden of the patenting process as far as formalities are concerned. Your company may have in-house staff specially qualified to deal with patents or those who are experienced in liason with external professional advisers. Because you are the inventor, however, it will be impossible to insulate you completely from the problems that arise if your company is patent-conscious and wishes to seek protection in your case. Your input of technical data and your understanding of the invention will be crucial to the outcome. Patenting is hardly ever a routine matter and various problems and objections have to be overcome in the process. You must expect to be involved in the explanation and defence of your invention and in distinguishing it from prior knowledge. If you are working in a research institution which is non-industrial the institution may well have a clear policy for patenting and exploitation of research results in which case you will not be totally free to put the matter into the hands of others. You or the institution may allow patenting to be undertaken by a selected industrial company or some other collaborating body but as the originator of the invention your continued participation is always desirable and often essential. In neither of the above situations will you be able to opt out altogether and it would be better to maintain some level of interest in what is done with your invention and how it is protected even though the experience may be rather strange at first.

10   Does a patent give me the right to put my invention into commercial use?

A patent does not convey this right in a positive sense. The inventor does not need a patent in order to be free to use his invention. This freedom itself stems from the freedom of enterprise which is enjoyed in most industrialised countries. Therefore it is qualified only by the pre-existing rights of others and also by any other laws which are relevant e.g. health and safety regulations. Thus a particular invention covered by a particular patent may be dominated by a prior patent of broader scope. The mutual impact between the earlier and the later patents requires legal analysis and often negotiation between the parties concerned to determine their respective rights and freedoms.

11   Is a patent territorially limited?

Yes because it is granted by the authority of a Department of State under the national law of that State and therefore its effect cannot normally extend beyond the jurisdiction of the latter.

12   What about 'world' patents?

There are no such thing. Prior to 1978 all patents were national patents limited in scope as stated above. In 1978 the European patent system came into practical operation as the first important example of a 'regional' patent. A European patent can cover a group of contracting States which are parties to the European Patent Convention. Even here, however, although the process of obtaining the European patent is a single centralised procedure, the final patent is not a single item of property but in effect a bundle of national patents (see Glossary, under European Patent Convention). The other form of international patent procedure is provided for under the Patent Co-operation Treaty but again the international aspect is of temporary duration covering only the early stages of patent procedure and in effect the international application separates into parallel national applications in the later stages.

13   One often sees equipment marked 'patent applied for' or 'patent' or even 'world patents pending'. What does this mean?

This marking deserves little attention unless specific patent application numbers or granted patent numbers are quoted in which case information can be found concerning the nature of the patent rights and whether they are still in force. By marking equipment in this way the proprietor intends to notify others that he owns or has applied for patent rights in certain countries. The object of marking products is to warn anyone thinking of copying them that they should beware of infringing the proprietor's rights. This is a genuine and valid legal custom carried out in the interests of the owner of the patent or potential patent. Sometimes the practice has little more than nuisance value because the patents may not have been granted or may never be granted or may have lapsed for one reason or another.

14   Are there industrial property rights other than patents?

There is a system for the registration of designs rather similar to the patent system. Registered designs are essentially concerned with features of shape, pattern and ornament. Therefore they are of primary interest for items of equipment such as furniture, fittings, boats, cars, etc., and they have little to do with the processes and products of biotechnology. Trade marks is the other major system of industrial property rights and these are of enormous commercial importance. A good trade mark coupled with a secret process of manufacture can be very valuable commercially, 'Coca-Cola' being an excellent example. Trade marks are essentially for those in trade and commerce and are therefore usually handled by the commercial business side of an organisation rather than being of central interest to the inventor or research worker. For new varieties of plants there is another legal system of protection which is similar to the patent system but distinct from it in some important respects. All the systems mentioned so far require positive action to register the claim. Copyright protection requires very little by way of registration and comes into being as soon as the author of the work has created it and recorded it in some suitable documentary form.

15   Does copyright law have any special application to biotechnology?

Micro-organisms and DNA sequences 'reproduce' and 'copy' themselves and there is a great temptation to apply these notions to the language of copyright law which seems to read precisely on to what happens in biological systems. Although some lawyers do pursue this question it is more commonly believed that it involves a false analogy and is likely to be a dead end as regards useful property rights. This question is dealt with in Appendix 2. For the present it should be noted that copyright protects only against direct copying and not against independent research. Moreover it is rather narrow protection in that there is no copyright in an underlying idea but only in its form or mode of expression.

16   Secrecy seems to be an alternative to patenting and involves less distraction from research work. Is this a viable option?

Patenting an invention or keeping it secret are incompatible options. Patents were invented in order to induce disclosure of new technology and thereby enable society to benefit from the knowledge of it as well as from the mere availability of it in the form of some product produced by a secret process. The Carthusian monks have kept secret for centuries the process of making Chartreuse without denying the benefit of it to mankind. For most research workers, who would find it difficult to keep a vow of perpetual silence, this option is unattractive.

An obvious first sub-division of attitudes on this question would be between the scientist working in an academic institution and an industrial research worker whose first loyalty is to his employer. Even here the distinction is not clear cut and each camp will break down into a range of opinions. The only certain conclusion at first glance is that if you are under pressure to publish you will need to consider very seriously the possibility of patent protection in your case. This question is dealt with further in Appendix 3.

17   How do I know if I have made an invention worth patenting?

Fortunately a good many research workers have an intuition which may prompt them to think about the practical applications of their work. A basic awareness of these possibilities has to be in the mind of the research worker in the first place and it is hoped that this and other elementary books about patents may help to create such awareness. There is no doubt that once you have broken the ice with the patenting of your first invention you will have become that much wiser for the future. Even if your first experience has proved rather frustrating and unsuccessful you should persevere in the knowledge that the field of innovation is inherently likely to result in a number of setbacks before the winner is achieved.

18   The word 'invention' sounds rather grand. What level of ingenuity is necessary for something to qualify as a patentable invention?

A further answer will be reserved until a later chapter in which the formal requirement of inventive step is discussed. For the present you should not be put off by the expression and give it too elevated an interpretation. The vast majority of inventions that are patented are a world apart from those that attract a Nobel prize; the criteria are quite obviously different. A whole spectrum exists ranging from radically new processes and products to relatively minor improvements in existing technology. There is, however, often no necessary correlation between high inventive achievement in the scientific and legal sense and commercial value and success.

A distinction is also to be made between invention and innovation. Innovation is the introduction of something as new and it has a practical connotation of 'getting things done' for the first time. Invention requires a stricter standard of novelty. Many innovations are impossible to patent because of this.

19   In considering patents what do I commit myself to as regards effort and expense?

Patenting involves a commitment if you want to see it through to the end. You can withdraw at any time if you are prepared to write off the expenditure entailed up to that point. However patenting is not a slot machine operation in which you simply insert the fee and take the product. It is essentially an adversarial process in which you will have to argue your case with Patent Office officials (examiners) and others. To obtain worthwhile results from the system you will have to understand the timescales and deadlines for taking certain action and producing certain data. You will be guided fully in these respects by professional advisors and others and it will be their job to bear most of the tedium. However you must be prepared to assist in the drafting of specifications and the preparation of arguments against the inevitable official objections that are raised during examination of your patent application.

20   Do I need a patent agent or can I do it all myself?

The answer is yes to both parts of this question. Having the help of someone skilled in patent law will not guarantee the absence of problems for the simple reason that in order to establish patentability there may be official objections which are difficult to overcome. Also your agent cannot deliver results if you have not done enough work on your invention to support the type and breadth of patent you would like to obtain. Doing it yourself on the other hand is almost certain to be disastrous except in the case of a simple invention in non-complex technology. You may receive sympathy and help from the Patent Office examiner but by the time he comes to examine your application it will be too late to add the necessary data to plug gaps in your patent

description or to enable you to make distinctions between your
invention and the prior art. Doing it yourself in this way suffers from the
lack of a professional critical approach to your data from the very
beginning which would have anticipated the critical treatment that the
examiner is obliged by law to give to your patent application.

In any event the DIY approach cannot be followed for foreign patents
and you will need a local agent in each foreign country for national
applications. You could file a DIY European patent application but the
chances are that you would soon find the formalities overwhelming and
would need a European patent attorney to help cope with the complex
regulations. The cost would also be formidable for the inventor without
significant financial resources.

21   Are there organisations that can help you with patents and exploitation?

For the private individual or research worker in a privately-funded or
publicly funded research institution there is now a fair number of
organisations that can help. They vary widely in character and in the
range of services offered. For example, the availability of funds for
extensive patenting and the even more costly operation of developing
promising but immature inventions is not uniform. One common feature
of all such organisations is that they will apply their critical faculty to the
ideas and research results you may have and they will inevitably be
selective in what they will support and finance.

The major organisations will not act as mere agencies or brokers but
will want to sit in the driving seat when it comes to exploitation. For this
they will need to have your rights assigned to them and the patents
eventually held in their name. Your name will be on the patent as
inventor and it will appear on the published patent specification. But it
must be stressed that there cannot be too many drivers if the
exploitation activity is to be conducted in a business-like manner. For
example licence negotiations cannot be efficiently run by a committee
and someone has to manage them even though consultation with the
inventor and his employing institution may be very desirable from time
to time.

Some of these organisations are national and public and have a remit
which reflects their origin and foundation. Most of them will
nevertheless attempt to operate internationally and cover the major
market areas in biotechnology. It should be possible to obtain
information about available organisations from official public sources
concerned with innovation, e.g. The Department of Trade and Industry
in the United Kingdom. One has to be careful about the stability and
professionalism of any of these organisations.

3   Avoiding the pitfalls

The consequences of ignorance of the patent law can be unfortunate for the inventor. Before approaching the ways in which patentability is dealt with according to objective criteria it is worth discussing first some of the more common ways in which inventors can themselves unwittingly undermine their position. It is essential to know the pitfalls and traps that must be avoided in the path leading up to the filing of a patent application. For lack of understanding of the way in which the novelty requirement in patent law is applied many an invention has lost the possibility of protection through prejudicial disclosure or use. All the questions dealt with in this chapter revolve around this central fact.

1   How much should I know about patents in order to get off to a proper start?

It is important to be aware of certain basic points of patent law to avoid making mistakes that can prove troublesome or disastrous later. The most common mistake is to be unaware that premature disclosure or use of an invention before the filing of any patent application may completely prejudice the chances of obtaining valid protection. Various kinds of prior disclosure or prior use of an invention in the pre-filing period will be identified and exemplified later.

2   Why should previous publication or use of my own work go against me when I start the patenting process?

Because the law requires that the invention is new at the time of filing the patent application. Most national patent laws use a definition of novelty which makes no distinction between your own prior disclosure and those of other workers. There are exceptions which will be mentioned later but the prevailing idea is that whatever is already in the public domain cannot be subsequently withdrawn by the inventor. The concept is that the grant of patent rights is a privilege rather than a basic right and it must therefore be conformed to certain rules which are believed to be in the public interest. Moreover the time for which the inventor's monopoly lasts is strictly limited. If an inventor were allowed to publish or otherwise disclose or exploit his invention in such a way as to establish scientific priority or commercial advantage and only later to decide to patent the invention there would be uncertainty for third parties which could work against the public interest. In any discussion about the legal philosophy of patents a fair balance must be struck between the inventor's rights and those of third parties. Under the law of the European Patent Convention, for example, the invention must be new over the 'state of the art' which is defined as

> 'everything made available to the public by means of a written or oral description, by use, or in any other way, before the date of filing of the European patent application'.

This requirement is referred to as 'absolute novelty'.

3   How much can I disclose without harming my future patent position?

The key concept here is one of a so-called 'enabling disclosure'. If the disclosure is such as to give the reader or recipient enough information to carry out the inventive process or make the inventive product or apparatus for himself then it can be extremely harmful if unprotected in any way. If more is necessary to achieve this than is contained in the disclosure e.g. if access is required to a non-available micro-organism strain or some other biological material then one can argue that the disclosure does not completely destroy novelty. However, the disclosure of the information might still be pertinent to the question of inventiveness.

Most disclosures which are made without thinking about patents will give enough information to practise the invention and this will certainly be harmful. The more indefinite the disclosure the more innocuous it is as regards subsequent patenting. For example a general reference to results obtained without saying precisely how they were or could be obtained may not be totally damaging. It will depend entirely on the circumstances and the safe advice is to think before you speak or write anything about your new ideas and results.

4   What are the exceptions to the general rule about prejudicial prior disclosure?

The exceptions are limited to those countries in which the national law provides for 'grace periods'. A grace period is a period of time immediately preceding the filing of a patent application during which public disclosure or use of one's own invention will not destroy the possibility of protection in a country that provides for a grace period. The most usual situation in which grace periods have to be invoked is that of an inventor who makes a literature publication or some other form of oral or written disclosure of his work and later wishes or is advised by others to seek patent protection. Protection will then be possible only in countries in which there is sufficient time to prepare and file the patent application before the grace period expires. The most important grace periods are those of the USA (1 year), Canada (2 years) and Japan (6 months under special conditions) but some other countries also provide them. More details of these are given in Appendix 4.

European patent law has no grace period for dealing with situations described above. However, the European Patent Convention provides a sort of grace period of 6 months which can be used where unauthorised publication of an inventor's work by some other party has taken place. This can happen through inadvertance or by actual breach of confidence. It is necessary to show that the publication occurred without the inventor's consent. Most other national laws in Europe which conform to the European Convention also have this feature.

5   **Are grace periods available to all inventors irrespective of nationality?**

Yes. The grace periods are limited to the national laws of the countries concerned but are not restricted to their own nationals, i.e. citizens or residents. If an inventor has unwittingly published his invention before taking thought about patenting then the US grace period provision is available to him irrespective of his nationality or location. Indeed many European inventors have benefited from the US grace period by rescuing a patent position in the USA after publication. The US inventor who has likewise published can also still obtain a US patent but in those countries where no grace period provisions exist his own publication will be considered as part of the state of the known art which is citable against him. It is also worth pointing out that the *place* where the disclosure is made is of no consequence in the law of the 'absolute novelty' countries.

Interferon was discovered in 1957 by research workers in Britain and was first isolated and shown by them to have properties as an antiviral agent. Before patent action was considered two articles appeared in Proceedings of the Royal Society *in September 1957. These would have been protected publications under the then prevailing British patent law i.e. exempted as publications in the transactions of a Learned Society. Unfortunately a leading article on interferon in the* British Medical Journal *was issued on November 1957 and put an end to the possibility of a British patent. However the grace periods of USA, Canada, and West Germany allowed the filing of patent applications in these countries and patents were granted. The United States patent (3,699,222) eventually issued in October 1972.*

6   **It still sounds complicated. If there is no uniformity of attitude
from country to country towards the prior publication or prior
use of my own work how can I cope with so many variations when
I decide to take the first step towards obtaining protection?**

You do not have to tackle everything at once. This will be made clear in
the next chapter dealing with the sequence of steps in the patenting
operation. Fortunately there is over a century of international
cooperation in patent law and there are a number of international
conventions which greatly simplify the handling of these matters. The
most helpful of all is the Paris Convention which allows an international
priority right to be given to your first patent application (which is usually
made in your country of residence). Consequently this allows you to
delay applying for foreign patents for a certain period without loss of
recognition of your priority. The Paris Convention and the availability of
grace periods in a few countries give rise to the possibility of a certain
amount of manipulation by expert hands to secure the desired result.

It must be said however that matters are much simplified if a research
worker is willing to suspend publication for a sufficient time (not too
great) to enable the patenting operation to be properly launched. The
industrially employed inventor is usually disposed to accept this
constraint in the interests of his employer and as a result industry does
not often need to make use of the grace periods for inventions made by
its own research staff.

7   **In spite of grace periods it seems that the research worker must
be very secretive about his work in the early stages. It may be
virtually impossible to maintain secrecy for more than a very
short time. Is there a solution to this problem?**

There are two main reasons for being prudent about disclosing new
discoveries at too early a stage. The first reason is that disclosure can
destroy the chances of obtaining useful protection in view of the
absolute novelty requirements of most patent laws and this has been
referred to above. A second reason is that industrial competitors or rival
research groups are put on notice of the direction of your research and
may in fact beat you to the post as regards patent priority and perhaps
even scientific priority. This second reason is already very familiar to
research workers who practise a considerable degree of reticence under
the increasing competitiveness of research in the academic world as well
as in other environments. Because of this the scientific worker should
not be entirely unreceptive to advice as to caution about the disclosure
of preliminary findings. For the present however it is only the first of
these reasons that will be dealt with.

The problem of maintaining secrecy can be exaggerated to the point at which one might despair of ever obtaining a valid patent. Such a pessimistic approach should be avoided. The problem should be patiently analysed in order to discover solutions best suited to the different ways in which it can arise in the circumstances of real life. Thus the disclosure can be oral or written, public or private, i.e. confidential, and there may be other distinctions which affect the legal conclusion. It is not always certain even to professionally qualified people whether a particular kind of disclosure would be held prejudicial in a court of law. It is best always to seek advice about a specific situation before ruling out the possibility of protection or before proceeding to embark on a costly patent programme which may turn out to be futile.

8   What is the difference in legal effect between an oral and a written disclosure prior to patenting?

The written disclosure is the most deadly form of prior disclosure, especially the literature publication or documentation distributed prior to oral presentation at a scientific meeting. The US and Japanese patent laws, for example, pay particular attention to whether or not the document is one for distribution or intended to be accessible to a range of interested people. Thus US patent law specifies 'printed publications' when dealing with prior disclosures which are a statutory bar to patentability but distribution or public access is the key note and the term 'printed' should not be taken too literally.

Oral disclosures can be equally deadly but it would be better to come to these after discussing a few more important points about written disclosure.

9   For journal articles what is taken to be the publication date?

A journal article will have a date of submission, date of acceptance, and date of issue of the journal. It has sometimes been argued that once an inventor has embarked on the process of publication the cat should be considered out of the bag from the first step and at least on the date of acceptance of the paper by the journal. However this argument has usually not succeeded and there is a general working consensus that the date on which the journal issues is the effective publication date for purposes of patent law. It is open to high level legal authority to decide this point specifically but probabilities are a guide to life.

In submitting an article to a journal an author intends it to go through the normal channels and procedures and he is entitled to assume until his paper appears in print that its confidentiality will have been respected. It cannot be assumed for legal purposes however that the actual publication date is the nominal issue date of the particular volume or number of the journal. There can be delays in distribution and sometimes there can be some circulation before the date shown on the front of the journal. From the strict legal view point the relevant date is that on which subscribers or other members of the public have actually received the information or can be assumed to have done so. It is therefore often necessary to check these facts with the publishers. In the best legal practice the burden of proof of effective publication date lies with the party asserting it although it is sometimes necessary for the applicant or patentee against which the publication is cited to go to some trouble to destroy the presumption of public availability of the document as of its nominal date. The same considerations apply to the publication of other kinds of document including patent specifications.

10   **Can I submit my communication or paper to a journal and use the residence time before actual publication in which to seek advice on patents?**

There are some risks in adopting this practice and it cannot be recommended as a rule. It is a compromise which can work in suitable circumstances. Various factors have to be considered. First, as indicated in the answer to question 9, it will be assumed that strict confidentiality attaches to your paper in the interim before actual publication. Accordingly the question of patenting has to be dealt with in the anticipated delay in processing of the paper by the journal. If your paper is particularly topical and nicely fills the gap in an issue being prepared for publication it may appear earlier than expected and you will have to beware of some surprises. Your patent advisers will need adequate time in which to prepare and file the patent application in the proper professional manner. In a race against a deadline some important points of appreciation may be missed by the patent agent and you may not spot the defect, unversed as you are in the drafting and interpretation of patents. A discussion between research worker and patent agent will often be necessary to bring out some important points that are lacking in the understanding of either party. If your agent has handled a fair number of inventions in your field of technology you may be surprised at his command of the background and his perspicacity when he interrogates you on key issues. But you cannot assume that he has had this experience and it may take a number of drafts and more than one discussion together before the specification is in the best possible shape to protect you properly.

A major drawback to this *fait accompli* approach is that the work you report in your paper may be insufficient to support patent cover of the broad scope necessary to give you solid protection. For example it may be necessary or at least very desirable to carry out some additional experiments to clarify certain technical points so that the inventive concept can be confidently defined in the application before your paper is published. If you are not disposed to do extra work you may have to accept a more limited scope of patent in these circumstances. But at least you should know the options and allow for possible reconsideration of the timing of your publication. There are some journals that will take a paper to the printer's proof stage and then hold it up awaiting clearance from the author to proceed. This will of course depend on the quantity of material the journal has for publication and one might not be able to rely on more than a few months of suspense in these circumstances.

11   **Do oral disclosures have a similar damaging effect if made prior to filing a patent application?**

In the patent laws of most countries an oral disclosure is in principle on the same footing as a written one. It follows that an oral disclosure which is made quite evidently for the purpose of freely transmitting knowledge about a new process, product, or whatever, is a gift to the public domain under any law having the same so-called 'absolute novelty' concept as the European law indicated above. In practice the oral disclosure may leave no trace if it is not subsequently written up as a record of what was said. It would therefore be inaccessible to the Patent Office examiner but would nevertheless remain lurking below the surface perhaps to be cited later by a third party as a reason for revoking or declaring invalid any patent obtained as a result of the examiner having been unaware of this item of prior art. It would then be a matter of proof by the testimony of one or more persons present as to what was disclosed on the particular occasion.

Oral disclosures are not so damaging under US patent law in which the conditions of novelty defined in the statute are expressed in terms of what is known to others through patents and other printed publications. In any case the US law has a one-year grace period which provides a fair margin of safety for disclosure by the inventor. Oral disclosures occur in a variety of circumstances and each should be considered separately.

> *Two United States Patents 4,189,534 and 4,293,654 covering cell culture micro carrier technology developed at the Massachusetts Institute of Technology (Levine et al.) were held invalid by the Court of Appeals for the Federal Circuit partly on account of prior disclosure at a scientific conference. A paper relevant to the inventions was presented orally by one of the inventors at the First International Cell Culture Congress in Birmingham, Alabama, more than one year before the patent applications*

were filed. Prior to the conference a copy of the paper was given to the organiser and afterwards copies were distributed to six persons without restriction also more than one year before filing. The argument that the paper was not a printed publication was rejected by the Court and the paper was held to be prior art citable against the two patents.

12   Reading a paper or making a statement at a scientific conference is presumably the most common example of oral disclosure?

It is indeed. Sometimes an academic worker may say 'I haven't published this yet but I did speak about it at the Helsinki meeting last year'. This implies a much too narrow view of the meaning of 'publish' as far as patent law is concerned. The reading of a paper, or even a statement made by a member of the audience, at conferences of this kind must be assumed to be a true public disclosure with the intention or at least the acceptance of the fact that the knowledge can be utilised by others. This assumption itself takes it for granted that the scientific meeting is a truly public gathering rather than the coming together of an elite to receive information in some privileged way.

13   What kinds of oral disclosure can be regarded as confidential?

Disclosure is confidential if (a) the person passing the information makes it clear that it is *intended* to be confidential and (b) it is evident that the disclosure is *in fact* confidential. Both conditions must be present. It is possible for a person to indicate an intention of confidentiality attaching to an oral or even a written disclosure and yet the circumstances are such that confidentiality is in fact incompatible with the nature of the disclosure. For example a report intended for distribution to members of an industrial research association so that it might be utilised in a practical and public way could not be saved from prejudicing later patenting simply by being stamped 'confidential to members only'.

Sometimes a disclosure can be considered to be confidential even without an explicit statement if the circumstances are such that confidentiality is implied.

14   Does patent law extend confidentiality to disclosures to colleagues in the laboratory or elsewhere in industrial establishments and in academic institutions?

Within an industrial environment discussions with colleagues on the subject of current research must be privileged and under commercial security. This would be the natural assumption within the research laboratory and it must also apply to disclosure to other departments. Universities and other like institutions obviously cannot be totally equated with industry for this purpose but even here there should be no question that discussions with research colleagues are privileged. But a variety of disclosures take place within an academic institutional setting and they cannot all be assumed to be entitled to exemption in this respect. If the meeting is a purely internal one it can be argued that the disclosure is private and not public because it is made to a special group who are under one employer or one allegiance. On the other hand if 'outsiders' are invited it becomes more difficult to argue that confidence is implicit especially if some of the invitees are from the commercial world. It would certainly help if an express statement of confidentiality were made at meetings of this sort at universities and elsewhere. The frequent difficulty here is to persuade the academic worker to think along these lines which are unfamiliar and sometimes felt to be alien to such scientists. Usually patent advice is not sought until after the meeting has taken place and the patent adviser is then often genuinely puzzled in attempting to assess whether the circumstances of the disclosure are such as to fall short of what the law would consider to be a truly public disclosure prejudicial to any subsequent attempt to seek patent protection. It must be stressed that there is little or no case law directly dealing with the special situation and problems of the academic worker and one therefore has to argue from first principles, as is clearly being done in the present answer.

15 **In universities meetings are often held which have a special character. For example the meeting may be for a limited audience selected from among the most outstanding workers in a particular field. The object of such a meeting will be to exchange information primarily for research purposes in order to advance a newly developing line of research perhaps more rapidly and effectively than by the normal processes of literature publication. It would therefore be primarily academic in motivation and not concerned with commercial application. What would the status of such meetings be according to patent law?**

Patent law makes no distinction between disclosures for academic purposes and those aimed at a commercial objective. It would be extremely difficult to lay down legal criteria for such a distinction. Moreover the distinction may not be valid anyway. Many important industrial processes and products are based on knowledge derived from academic publication and in the present era when new industrial technology is essentially research-based the academic worker can no longer remain isolated from the commercial implications of his research. Moreover the context of this question is one in which the academic worker subsequently wants to patent his work and so it becomes difficult to maintain the distinction proposed. The only real solution here would be to provide for a grace period under international law.

But the situation may not be entirely hopeless. Provided such meetings are of a special and privileged character there is nothing to stop any participant from stating that certain parts of his oral presentation are sensitive, are likely to be the subject of a patent application in the near future, and are therefore disclosed as advance information which can be noted but not freely utilised. Of course this is to tread a thin line and there is no guarantee that it is legally secure. It is a last-resort piece of advice when there is insufficient time before the meeting to prepare and file a patent application. The form of confidentiality statement is best checked with the patent agent first. If the inventor can be induced to take this precaution it is but a short step for him in future to notify a patent expert in time to enable an application to be filed in advance!

The closed workshop is an example of the type of meeting under discussion here. One has to be wary of the consequences of pre-circulation of printed papers or abstracts to the participants. These should preferably be marked as confidential by the organisers (or authors) in case they become available later to individuals who might otherwise assume that the document constitutes an open publication. This would then put the burden of proof on the inventors to show that the disclosure was in fact confidential.

16   **It is often necessary to make reports or propose a programme of work to various committees, official bodies and other bodies. Is this confidential?**

Reports to official bodies or proposals made to funding organisations are presumed to be in confidence at least in the early stages of consideration, refereeing etc. If at some later stage it becomes necessary to publish the information openly or distribute it rather widely it will have been necessary in the meantime to take whatever protective action is possible on the data available.

A proposal for supporting a programme of work from public sector sources of funds may be based on research data already obtained, which may or may not be sufficient for patent purposes. If a patentable invention has already materialised it would be best not to delay seeking protection. Even if no work has yet been done the idea behind the proposal may itself be part of the total inventive step and if there is any risk of unprotected disclosure this might prejudice future prospects of patent cover. It is difficult to say more than this except in specific cases where the paper or proposal can be vetted professionally in this respect.

Disclosures to private sector organisations are probably less clear cut. Venture capital organisations and similar bodies are quite ready to receive proposals for evaluation and to give to them as much confidentiality as is consistent with their need to obtain impartial advice on technical and commercial aspects. Industrial sponsors however are more cagey about disclosure in confidence because the acceptance of a confidential relationship may put them at a disadvantage in relation to on-going work in their own research laboratories.

17   **The answer to the previous question appears to pose a problem. The research worker may not be able to take effective action on the basis of preliminary results and yet he may have to disclose these in order to attract financial support. Is this not a real dilemma?**

It would clearly be absurd to encourage inventors to rush to the PatentOffice with premature ideas and therefore some working strategy must be developed to deal with the apparent dilemma. Awareness of the existence of this problem can go part of the way towards solving it. If the research has proceeded to a point at which something protectable by patents has emerged it is obviously better to file a patent application before making any disclosure which cannot be safely treated as privileged. It is in any case good policy to file a patent application in order to identify the rights which the inventors believe they are entitled to before any potential collaborator or third parties are brought in. If this is not possible and it is necessary to have outside collaboration before the emerging new technology is perfected to the point at which an invention can be defined then the collaboration should be set up on the basis of proper understanding of the obligations and expectations of the parties. Certainly the obligation of non-disclosure to others must be spelt out. The question of ownership of patent rights must also be frankly faced as well as the related issues of responsibility for exploitation of research results, the mechanism by which this is to be achieved, and the basis on which the proceeds are to be shared or used. A particular question under these headings arises from the possibility of joint inventive contributions from different members of the total team (inventorship problems will be the subject of another chapter). Working out a plan of this sort has the corollary that a considered approach to the choice of a scientific collaborator or a source of funds has been made. Hawking the idea around to different people and organisations in rapid succession (or even at the same time!) is not compatible with the structured approach and in any case it runs the risk of being viewed as a public disclosure activity.

To go further into this subject would take us into the items that should be covered in collaboration agreements or joint research projects. These can become rather complex and are best prepared by lawyers and therefore cannot be adequately covered in this discussion.

18   If I have to disclose information to other scientists or organisations whose help I may need e.g. for biological testing how should I do so?

Sending out samples of new chemical compounds or other biological material for biological activity screening and other tests is not uncommon and it is the general understanding that these exchanges of information and material are privileged. Sending material out under a code name is the natural solution from the patent law view point but the recipient may not be prepared to accept the material without some indication of composition or origin. There is no patent law difficulty about some limited form of disclosure in these circumstances provided there is no doubt as to its confidentiality. Even disclosing the total identity of the material to be tested will not be held to be publication in these circumstances. Preferably all unused material should be returned or destroyed after the tests are completed.

If the supplier of the material suggests the type of screen he requires, because he already has some idea of the type of activity the material may have, there is no possibility of a co-inventorship situation arising between the supplier and the person running the tests. If however the latter has the bright idea of testing for a rather unusual activity and one that has not been suggested or implied by the supplier this could give rise to an additional invention beyond that of the material *per se* i.e. a further biological application of the material. Such a development would not necessarily be unwelcome but ought at least to be contemplated beforehand.

19   Suppose it is necessary to seek outside help for the structural chemical characterisation of a new compound?

It is sometimes necessary to send out uncharacterised or partially characterised material for spectral determinations which throw light on chemical structure or which even fingerprint the molecule. The characterisation of new products by spectral data is a legitimate means of defining a compound for the purposes of a patent although if a chemical formula can be assigned to the material so much the better. It is clear that sending out pure material for characterisation does not count as a public disclosure and therefore provided the usual precautions as to secrecy are understood and maintained the inventor's position is in no way endangered. Furthermore, in the view of the writer, analytical work of this kind however skilful does not in itself give the analyst any legal claim to co-invention of the compound and it is fortunately rare for such a claim to be made. It is customary to acknowledge help of this kind in a scientific publication and occasionally it may justify co-authorship on the part of the analytical chemist but this is quite different from inventorship according to patent law.

20   **How does the prior use of an invention prejudice its patentability?**

A prejudicial prior use is one which makes the invention available to the public. For example US patent law refers specifically to 'public use' and any such use occurring in the USA more than one year before the US application is filed will be a bar to patentability. A sale of a product in the USA is on the same footing as public use. Public use or sale outside the USA is not considered prejudicial. European law indicates that making the invention publicly available by use before the patent application date (or priority date) means that it has become part of the state of the art and is therefore unpatentable. Public use anywhere in the world is prejudicial as regards the European Patent Convention.

21   **What is the position with regard to experimental use?**

Experimental use of an invention in the research laboratory or in the field is a necessary part of the entire process of making and evaluating an invention. Clearly this kind of use is not what the law would hold to be prejudicial. It has to be postulated of course that the experimental use is carried out under conditions of secrecy or strict confidentiality so that it does not constitute a public *disclosure* as such. Experimental use of this kind is not a public use because it is not intended to make anything available to the public yet and it does not do so in fact. So far so good. There will come a point when the making and evaluating of the invention are sufficiently advanced to enable the question of patent protection to be considered. The cautious inventor may still feel that a further trial period is necessary before making a commitment to spend money on patenting and to the writing of a specification which will not have to be radically changed next week because of developments. Further trials for a short period of a few months or more would be regarded as within the category of experimental use.

Under present European law once the experimental and reasonable trial stages have been completed it is time to consider the situation carefully. If the inventor then starts to put the invention into routine use and the circumstances are such that other persons become aware of this use without any restriction it would invalidate a subsequent application. If however the routine use is carried out in secret it may be that nothing at all becomes available to the public. For example if the invention is an item of laboratory apparatus and no visitors are ever allowed into the laboratory it is difficult to see what has been made available to the public. Whilst an element of uncertainty may be present in circumstances of this latter kind from which advantage may possibly be taken the recommended action is always to apply for a patent for putting an invention into routine use of any kind.

22   **Can prior use of an invention before seeking patent protection be harmful if it takes place without knowledge of the invention passing into the public domain?**

A general answer cannot be given to this question as there may well be differences in the views of courts of law in different countries. This point has not yet been raised as a matter of interpretation of European patent law or of any national laws which have the same definition of the state of the art. However under the British patent law existing before 1977 the English courts dismissed the idea that knowledge must pass before the prior use could be held prejudicial. Most of the decided cases were concerned with prior use of a kind which amounted to an attempt to exploit and benefit from an invention before applying for a patent, e.g. to secure an order for the purchase of equipment. In the latest such case decided under the old British law the argument that the sales promotion activity was confidential and involved no supply of information about what was in the 'black box' being offered for sale was rejected by the court and the patent held invalid. It is not certain that the courts of other countries would take the same position as the British judges or indeed that this position will remain unchanged under the present law.

For the industrial worker in a company that may not be properly aware of the legal complications the main danger may be that of publicity for the purposes of marketing and actual use of an invention for production and sale prior to filing a patent application. For the non-industrial worker it would be useful to pin up a notice in the laboratory showing the proper order of events:

INCEPTION – RESEARCH – INVENTION –
DEVELOPMENT– PUBLICITY– EXPLOITATION

into which PATENTING must be inserted somewhere between INVENTION and PUBLICITY.

In dealing with pitfalls of this kind we have excluded the situation where a grace period can be utilised. Since grace periods are the exception it is better for the inventor to become adapted to the more regular environment. There is a significant body of opinion in favour of making grace periods the rule rather than the exception but this would require a major international effort and a legal change of this kind could not be achieved quickly.

23   **It seems that publication by others will prevent me getting a patent even though I did the work before the publication appeared. Are there exceptions to this rule?**

The most important exceptions are the laws of USA and Canada which do take into account the date of actual invention as well as the date of filing a patent application. A simplified statement of the US law relevant to this particular question is that the novelty requirement is met so long as the invention was:

(a)   not known or used by others in USA   before the applicant's
                      or   *invention* date
       not described in a printed publication

and

(b)   not described in a printed publication   more than 1 year before
                      or   the applicant's US
       not in public use or on sale in USA   *filing* date.

Proviso (a) introduces the concept of invention date as distinct from filing date and hence the US law is called a 'first-to-invent' system as contrasted with the 'first-to-file' system of most other countries. An inventor can establish an invention date by means of laboratory notebook or other records held in USA to show conception and reduction to practice of an invention at a date significantly earlier than his patent application date. This facility, which is known as 'swearing back' can enable the inventor to avoid the otherwise damaging effect of the other person's prior publication. However, the inventor cannot delay filing his patent application for too long because after one year the prior publication becomes a 'statutory bar' under proviso (b) above.

Where the prior publication is authored by the inventor himself, proviso (b) is the basis for the grace period mentioned earlier in this chapter. Where the publication is by another person it can therefore only be overcome if the inventor can establish an earlier invention date and has filed a US application within one year of the publication.

It cannot be emphasised too strongly that the swearing back facility applies only to inventions made in or introduced to the USA. The resident US inventor will take advantage of this by recording his 'invention disclosure' in writing and having it dated and witnessed by someone who states that he has read and understood it. The foreign inventor's record in his home country is of no avail for this purpose and must be sent to someone in USA for recording there. US attorney firms provide this service and keep records for production later if necessary either to overcome a Patent Office objection or in a dispute over priority of invention. Many non-US inventors and companies make regular use of this device and send memoranda or research reports to their US attorneys long before they have been processed for filing patent applications in their home country.

The Canadian system is similar to the US except in this important last respect that notebook evidence in the home country of the foreign inventor can establish invention date without the need to introduce it into Canada.

Note added in proof:
Canada has recently changed its law to move to a first-to-file system and to reduce the grace period to 1 year as well as making other changes.

4   Starting the patenting process

Previous chapters have identified basic principles and the precautions a
research worker must take in order to avoid a false start or an early
disaster. He who begins well has completed half the work and this is
particularly true of patenting as will soon appear. The writing of the
patent specification is the principal single act upon which all depends
and to do this well involves having a fair appreciation of the novelty of
the invention and its distinction from prior art. Secondly the
experimental ground must have been well covered and supporting data
must be available. Thirdly it must be clear which members of the
research team qualify as inventors in the true legal sense of the term as
these must be named either at the outset or a little later on in patent
proceedings. A typical dialogue on these themes follows.

1   **When and how does one start the patenting process?**

The motivation to begin this process normally comes from the inventor
as the generator of the ideas and results. If the inventor does not
recognise his opportunity and there is no other 'spotter' in the
organisation where the research is done then the opportunity may easily
slip away. There is a point to be struck between starting too early and
starting late. Of the two it is much better to take advice in the earlier
stages especially as this may direct the research into more productive
lines as regards patent protection. You should explain to your selected
adviser or confidant what your research is about, and its aims and its
achievements so far in terms of actual data. You should not assume that
he will already be fully abreast of your subject. The right time to start
patenting is when you have obtained sufficient data to formulate the
invention you want to protect. A conversation with a patent agent or
some other person with knowledge or experience of patenting will draw
out the factors to be considered. For example, an inventor will
sometimes focus too narrowly on immediate objectives and may not see
other applications of the research. A detached person with a fresh mind
can be of great help in correcting this.

2   **Since priority is very important how can it ever be too early to start?**

In patent terms it is of little use being first in the field, i.e. having the earliest priority date, if the content of your application is inadequate to achieve the broad scope of patent you might otherwise expect to obtain. There are at least two snags to filing a patent application too soon. The first is that the full scope or limitations of the invention may not be fully understood (by you) if the experimental evidence is still at an early stage. As the research proceeds it may be realised that the invention is not of such broad scope as first thought, in which case a more limited statement or claim will be necessary. Subsequent amendment of a patent application to limit the scope of a claim is possible and presents no problem so long as the basis for it can be found in the specification as filed. One cannot introduce arbitrary language to make an amendment. The second snag arises from the alternative possibility that further research shows the original specification to have been too narrowly worded. Additional data may now exist which would support a broader claim than was first envisaged. Once filed, an application cannot be expanded by the incorporation of new data because in patent language this is rejected as 'new matter'. The only way of broadening the protection in these circumstances is by means of another application; whether a further application is effective to achieve this objective depends on various factors which can only be properly assessed in the context of a particular case.

3   **Can I begin to patent with the basic idea alone?**

Invention may lie in the idea or in the way the idea is converted into practice or in the combination of the two. The United States patent law considers invention as involving the stage of 'conception' followed by that of 'reduction to practice'. The legal meaning of these terms is the subject of a fair amount of case law and cannot be fully explained here. However the ordinary meaning of these words is a simple starting point. Conception is the mental part of an invention and reduction to practice signifies either the experimental verification of the idea or the designing of some embodiment of it.

There is a difference here between inventing in the natural sciences and inventing in engineering. The engineer can take the conception stage towards some form of reduction to practice simply by making a design drawing, for example, of a mechanical device or an electrical circuit. Assuming that when it is subsequently constructed ('actual reduction to practice') the device or circuit behaves as expected then the invention will have been sufficiently complete for patent purposes even before the construction of the hardware. The chemist, on the other hand, may conceive of a chemical compound in terms of a structure which may be responsible for a particular biological activity but it will be necessary at least to prepare the compound before achieving reduction to practice. Even then it will be necessary for some testing to be done before the inventive act is considered complete. For a chemical or microbiological process it will be difficult to write a description of a reproducible process without there having been actual performance even if only on a laboratory scale.

For the biotechnology inventor it is best to assume that not much of a patent will be obtained without a reasonable amount of data from actual experiments.

4 **How can I assess the point at which my research is ready for an investigation of patentability?**

It would be helpful to have made some acquaintance with actual examples of patents to see how previous inventors have fared and the sort of data that have been considered sufficient to persuade a Patent Office to grant a patent. Apart from the basic question of novelty a useful test to apply would be to see whether you can write a description of the invention which, as far as content goes, compares with the patent specifications you have read. You can trace some of these by number in the various collections of Abstracts that are published e.g. Chemical Abstracts, but the best way would be to visit your National Patent Office or a library in any of the major cities that has collections of patents and simply browse through patents published in your field of interest.

Many patents are lengthy and complex but the following example of a US patent for a mutant strain of mushroom may be helpful as illustration (Figs. 4.1–4.7). Usually photographs are not included in specifications of microbiological invention, but in this case it was thought desirable to provide them.

5 **Some patents seem to have been obtained on very flimsy scientific evidence and questionable supporting data. These are obviously totally bogus. How do you account for this?**

The patent system is not perfect. It is difficult to give a completely satisfactory answer to this question but the following observations may help.

There are differences in the quality of examination of patent applications from one country to another and also from one Examiner to another in any single Patent Office. In certain countries there is no official criticism or examination of any kind and the patent is granted in

United States Patent [19]

Elliott et al.

[11]	**Patent Number:** **4,608,775**
[45]	**Date of Patent:** **Sep. 2, 1986**

[54] **MUSHROOM MUTANT STRAINS**

[75] Inventors: **Timothy J. Elliott**, Littlehampton; **Michael P. Challen**, Midhurst, both of England

[73] Assignee: **National Research Development Corporation**, London, England

[21] Appl. No.: **634,158**

[22] Filed: **Jul. 25, 1984**

[30]   **Foreign Application Priority Data**

Jul. 29, 1983 [GB]   United Kingdom 8320535

[51] **Int. Cl.⁴** **A01H 15/00**

[52] **U.S. Cl.** ....,............................. **47/1 R; 47/1.1; Plt./89**

[58] **Field of Search** 47/58, 1.1, 1; Plt./89

[56]   **References Cited**

PUBLICATIONS

T. J. Elliott and F. A. Langton, "Strain Improvement in the Cultivated Mushroom *Agaricus bisporus*", Euphytica 30, (1981), pp. 175–182.
"Mitteilung en der Versuchsanstalt fuer Pilzanbau der Landwirt Schaftskammer Rheinland Krefeld-Grossheuttenhof", Nov. 6, 1982, pp. 30–46 (English), article by T. J. Elliott.

Primary Examiner—Robert E. Bagwill
Attorney, Agent, or Firm—Murray and Whisenhunt

[57]   **ABSTRACT**

Sensitivity (lack of resistance) to fungicides is a problem in commercial strains of the mushroom *Agaricus bisporus*. Mutant strains, produced from the known parent strains by UV irradiation followed by selection, and having a genetically stable phenotype of insensitivity (resistance) to carboxin or benodanil have now been prepared. These mutant strains give a good yield of fruit in the presence of the fungicide. They have been deposited as patent deposits under the Budapest Treaty at the Commonwealth Mycological Institute.

7 Claims, 4 Drawing Figures

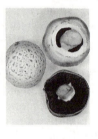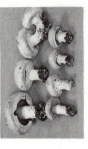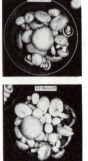

Fig. 4.1.

the form in which it has been written by the applicant. Consequently the validity of these patents is always questionable and it often requires court proceedings to determine just what scope of patent, if any, is sustainable. In the strict examination countries the Examiner has to be satisfied that a novel, inventive and practically applicable process or product is described in the specification before he can accept the application. There is an element of subjectivity therefore in what is considered by particular Examiners as meeting requirements. Also Examiners have to cover a wide field of subject matter and cannot know the prior literature in depth for every part of the field. Dubious patents must therefore be expected to appear sometimes.

The Examiner is not strictly obliged to consider the question of scientific proof or scientific evidence as such. Unless he can give good

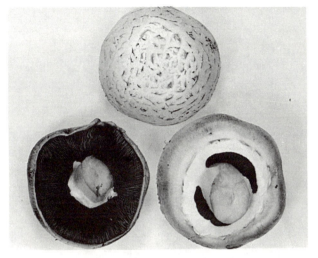

Fig. 1

Fig. 4.2.

reasons for suspecting the reliability of the applicant's data the Examiner (and the inventor's patent agent also) will accept the inventor's account as written in good faith. The applicant may be mistaken in his theory or the conclusions to be drawn from the data but the data as such are not usually challenged at this stage. Moreover an error of theory may not invalidate a patent so long as the process or product works and produces a useful result. Incidentally what appears to the scientist as a good reason against granting a patent may not be a good reason in law. Alternatively it may be one that cannot be brought within the terms of the allowed grounds of objection which can be raised by the Examiner. The Examiner ought to object if the description and data do not support or are not commensurate with the sort of patent being requested by the applicant and one is sometimes surprised by what passes through to

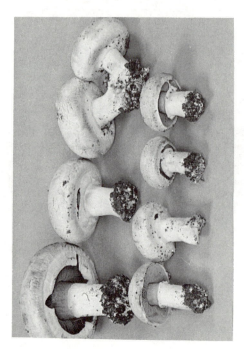

Fig. 4.3.

acceptance. The mere grant of a patent does not mean that the patent is valid and will withstand challenge from competitors and other third parties who may be in a position to attack the patent more cogently and severely and may have a strong motivation to do so.

In conclusion if you want a patent that is worth having do not be misled by the exceptions which get through the system. These are often a nuisance and therefore have a 'nuisance-value' to their owners but this is an illusion when the time of testing arrives. To build on a foundation of solid data is much the better course.

U.S. Patent   Sep. 2, 1986   Sheet 3 of 3   **4.608,775**

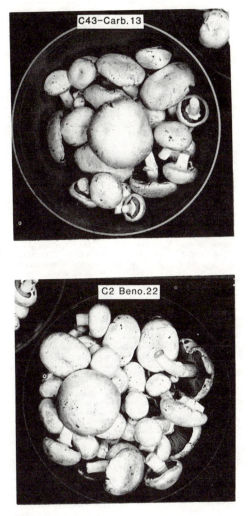

Fig. 4.4.

6   Should I try to write the patent specification?

As the inventor you are not expected to write the specification but it
will help your professional adviser enormously if you know the type of
information he will need and you write it up in the logical order in which
patent specifications are usually constructed.

4,608,775

1

MUSHROOM MUTANT STRAINS

This invention relates to new, fungicide-resistant strains of the mushroom *Agaricus bisporus*.

The fungus *Verticillium fungicola* is pathogenic to mushrooms and is troublesome to control. Certain fungicides, notably carboxin and benodanil, give some control over this pathogen, but these fungicides are phytotoxic to mushroom mycelium. If mushroom strains could be made less sensitive to one of these fungicides, the fungicide could be used to control fungal disease to which they are susceptible.

The mushroom *Agaricus bisporus* is a 2-spored species. That is, it has 2 spores on each basidium. The basidium contains a nucleus formed by fusion of two different but sexually compatible types of nuclei, i.e. carrying different genetic information. Call the nuclear types A and B. The basidium containing the nucleus AB undergoes meiosis to produce 2 spores per basidium. Each spore contains two nuclei and the predominant kind of spore is that containing the different compatible nuclei A and B. These spores therefore give rise to a self-fertile mushroom, since the A and B nuclei in the predominant spores fuse together to give a new nucleus within the basidium. There is therefore, natural in-breeding in *Agaricus bisporus*.

In commerce, it is usual to try to improve strains by selection from multi-spore cultures. This is an empirical approach and one which has not led to a great advance.

A more scientific way of producing strain improvement arises from occasional aberrance from 2 spore production. When occasionally 3 or 4 spores are produced, some of them inevitably contain only one nucleus (since the 4 nuclei produced by meiosis are shared between available spores). The mononucleate spores are not self-fertile: they need to fuse with other mononucleate spores to generate a pair of sexually compatible nuclei in the cells of the mycelium from which a new basidium is formed. Single spore cultures from aberrant basidia are therefore fused in order to generate new strains. The chances of improving the strain for any particular characteristic by this method are very low and, so far as is known, it has not resulted in an improvement in fungicide resistance.

The present invention is based on the mutation of commercially available strains of *Agaricus bisporus*, by irradiation, followed by a selection procedure to give new strains having reduced sensitivity (increased resistance) to carboxin or benodanil. The strains are self-fertile and their fungicide resistance phenotypes are genetically stable. Accordingly, the invention provides these mutant strains, samples of which have been deposited as patent deposits under the Budapest Treaty on the International Recognition of the Deposit of Microorganisms for Patent Purposes at the Commonwealth Mycological Institute, Ferry Lane, Kew, Surrey TW9 3AF, England, on July 9, 1984 under Accession Numbers 287345, 287343, 287344, and 287342. It also includes mutants and variants of each deposited strain.

Full particulars of the deposited mutant strains of the invention are as follows:

Parent strain from which derived	Deposit number at the CMI	Fungicide resistance phenotype	Sporophore character
"Somycel 11"	IMI 287345	Carboxin	Rough cap

Fig. 4.5.

2

-continued

Parent strain from which derived	Deposit number at the CMI	Fungicide resistance phenotype	Sporophore character
"Somycel 11"	IMI 287343	Carboxin resistance	Rough cap
"Darlington 649"	IMI 287344	Carboxin resistance	Smooth cap
"Mount White"	IMI 287342	Benodanil resistance	Smooth cap

The parent strains from which the mutants are derived are those produced by commercial mushroom spawn makers and in addition are available from the Glasshouse Crops Research Institute (an institute funded by the UK Government through the Agricultural and Food Research Council), Worthing Road, Littlehampton, West Sussex BN17 6LP, England.

The deposit IMI 287345 is the same as the deposit CMI CC 279364 made at the Commonwealth Mycological Institute on 25th July 1983, in connection with the UK Patent Application 8320535 from which priority is claimed, the sample or a sub-culture thereof having been transferred within the collection from U.K. national patent deposit to Budapest Treaty deposit status on 9th July 1984.

Mushrooms are classified according to whether their sporophores have smooth caps (which are usual in the UK) or rough caps. The rough caps have scales and are more off-white in appearance. (The character of the cap is affected by airflow and humidity, i.e. with high airflow and low humidity the amount of scaling increases).

The mushrooms produced by the mutants are of a quality comparable to those produced by their parents.

The invention includes a spawn comprising cereal grains, for example of rye, wheat or millet, and an *Agaricus bisporus* mutant strain of the invention. The formulation can be conventional and can therefore include also gypsum and calcium carbonate to improve flow characteristics and adjust the pH.

The invention is illustrated by the following description of the mutant strain IMI 287345 (previously CMI CC 279364).

The mycelium of the parent strain makes no growth on the medium containing more than 5–10 micrograms/ml of carboxin, i.e., its M.I.C. is 5–10 micrograms/ml. By contrast, the mutant strain IMI 287345 grows in the presence of more than 25 micrograms/ml of carboxin, i.e. its M.I.C. is 25–50 micrograms/ml. It is interesting to note that parent and mutant have a similar ED_{50} for carboxin, ED_{50} being the concentration of fungicide which restricts the radial growth of the mycelium by 50%. For the parent it is about 4 and for mutant about 5 micrograms/ml. Clearly, the mutant is capable of making slow growth at higher concentrations of carboxin than 4 micrograms/ml, whereas the growth of the parent falls to zero very sharply above this concentration.

Merely to find a mutant strain which is carboxin-resistant is not enough. It has to be one which grows well in the absence of carboxin. These two requirements are not very compatible. The mutant strain IMI 287345, however, does have the advantage of growing markedly better than its parent in the absence of carboxin, at the rate of 5.5 mm/day compared with 1.8 mm/day for the parent, as shown by in vitro tests.

4,608,775

3

The mutant strain is self-fertile, which suggests that it is heteroallelic for mating type, i.e. that the binucleate spores produced following meiosis contain different, compatible nuclei.

The genetic segregation of carboxin resistance of this mutant strain has been tested in the basidiospore progeny of a single spore. The pattern of carboxin-resistant phenotypes was consistent with there being a single dominant gene for carboxin resistance.

The fruiting ability of this mutant strain and its parent has been assessed in the presence and absence of carboxin. The mutant strain has consistently outyielded its parent and has maintained high productivity at concentrations of carboxin which reduce the yield of the parent by 30%.

In a trial of this mutant strain artificially infected with the mushroom pathogen *Verticillium fungicola* there was less disease in the fungicide-treated plots without concomitant loss of yield due to the phytotoxicity of carboxin.

The other strains of the invention are generally of a similar character, differing in their cap and in their precise degree and/or kind of fungicide resistance. They have shown good yields of fruit combined with good resistance to the fungicide. Thus IMI 287343 was found to be about 20% more productive than its parent strain and had an ED_{50} for carboxin of 20–25 micrograms/ml. IMI 287344 was about 5% more productive than its parent and had an ED_{50} for carboxin of 5–10 micrograms/ml, and an M.I.C. of 75–100 micrograms/ml, whereas the parent strain had the same ED_{50} but an M.I.C. of 15 micrograms/ml. IMI 287342 also yielded well in trials and had an ED_{50} for benodanil of between 10 and 20 micrograms/ml, and an M.I.C. of 50–75 micrograms/ml, whereas the parent strain had an ED_{50} of less than 5 and an M.I.C. of less than 10 micrograms/ml.

The general method of preparation of the deposited mutant strains comprises mutating the parent strain by UV irradiation, growing colonies of the irradiated strain on a medium containing the fungicide and subjecting the growing colonies to a growth procedure for selecting stable resistance to the fungicide. It must be emphasised, however, that this is not a recipe for quick success. The chances of obtaining a genetically stable fungicide resistant strain by the methods described are low (fewer than 1 in 300,000 of the original hyphal fragments typically survive and show the desired fungicide resistance) 1–2%, and the work is technically difficult. The particular method used is described below, using the induction of carboxin resistance as an example.

The parental strain was grown on complete yeast medium (hereinafter "CYM"), prepared as described below, until the colony fully covered the surface of the plate. Uniform agar plugs were cut from the plates and placed in sterile saline (8.1 g/liter) with a few drops of "Tween 80" as a wetting agent. ("Tween" is a Registered Trade Mark). Plugs and mycelium were macerated using a laboratory homogeniser. Aliquots of the homogenate were subjected to method (a) or (b) below for producing the mutants.

METHOD (a)

The homogenate was plated on solid CYM containing 15 micrograms/ml of carboxin. This concentration of carboxin was used in all carboxin-containing media in this method and in method (b). The plated material was irradiated for 10 seconds using UV light. The UV light

4

used had a wavelength of about 2537 Angstrom units, being the theoretical output of the lamp used.

The irradiated mycelium was incubated at 25° C. for 2–3 weeks. Only about 1% of the material showed growth. Visible mycelial colonies were transferred to a fresh solid CYM containing carboxin. The growing mycelium was then re-plated on solid CYM without fungicide and transferred to fresh solid CYM containing carboxin. This procedure selects only strains in which the carboxin resistance is stable as a result of induced mutation. Material in which the carboxin resistance is the result of physiological adaptation is unselected, as its progeny will not grow on the fresh fungicide medium.

METHOD (b)

The homogenate was plated into empty sterile petri dishes and irradiated for 10 seconds using UV light as in Method (a). The material was then transferred to liquid CYM containing carboxin. Flasks were intermittently shaken to increase aeration. The incubation temperature was 20°–25° C. (room temperature) and the time about 2 weeks. The growing mycelium was transferred to solid CYM containing carboxin. To select for stable carboxin resistance, the same procedure was used as in method (a).

Complete yeast extract (CYM) was prepared by autoclaving the following composition for 20 minutes at 121° C., and 2 atmospheres absolute pressure.

Ingredients	Grams/liter of distilled water
Peptone	2
Yeast extract	2
Glucose	20
Magnesium sulphate ($MgSO_4.7H_2O$)	0.5
Potassium dihydrogen phosphate	0.46
Dipotassium hydrogen phosphate and, when a solid medium is required:	1.0
Agar	20

The invention includes mutant and variant strains, especially those which give rise to stable resistance to the relevant fungicide, and, of course, subject to their giving rise to edible fruit. Preferred mutants and variants of the deposited strains include those conferring improved yield of fruit over the parent strains of the deposited strains, i.e. over "Somycel 11", "Darlington 649" and "Mount White". Mutants can be made by UV-irradiation or by the use of well known chemical mutagens. Variants can be made by breeding, including from aberrant basidia as described above in connection with the prior art.

BRIEF DESCRIPTION OF THE DRAWINGS

FIGS. **1** to **4** show fruit-bodies of *Agaricus bisporus* strains IMI 287345, 287343, 287344 and 287342 respectively.

We claim:

1. A biologically pure culture of a strain of *Agaricus bisporus* selected from the group consisting of the *Agaricus bisporus* strains IMI 287345, 287343, 287344 and 287342 deposited on 9th July 1984 at the Commonwealth Mycological Institute, Ferry Lane, Kew, Surrey TW9 3AF, England, under the provisions of the Budapest Treaty on the International Recognition of the Deposit of Micro-organisms for Patent Purposes.

Fig. 4.6.

4,608,775

5

2. A spawn composition comprising cereal grain and mycelium of an *Agaricus bisporus* strain specified in claim **1**.

3. Whole mushrooms derived from a culture of a strain of *Agaricus bisporus* selected from the group consisting of the *Agaricus bisporus* strains IMI 287345,287343,287344 and 287342 deposited on 9th July 1984 at the Commonwealth Mycological Institute, Ferry Lane, Kew, Surrey TW9 3AF, England, under the provisions of the Budapest Treaty on the International Recognition of the Deposit of Microorganisms for Patent Purposes.

4. *Agaricus bisporus* strain IMI 287345, deposited on 9th July 1984 at the Commonwealth Mycological Institute, Ferry Lane, Kew, Surrey, TW9 3AS, England, under the provisions of the Budapest Treaty on the International Recognition of the Deposit of Microorganisms for Patent Purposes.

6

5. *Agaricus bisporus* IMI 287343 deposited on 9th July 1984 at the Commonwealth Mycological Institute, Ferry Lane, Kew, Surrey, TW9 3AS, England, under the provisions of the Budapest Treaty on the International Recognition of the Deposit of Micro-organisms for Patent Purposes.

6. *Agaricus bisporus* strain IMI 287344 deposited on 9th July 1984 at the Commonwealth Mycological Institute, Ferry Lane, Kew, Surrey, TW9 3AS, England, under the provisions of the Budapest Treaty on the International Recognition of the Deposit of Micro-organisms for Patent Purposes.

7. *Agaricus bisporus* strain IMI 287342 deposited on 9th July 1984 at the Commonwealth Mycological Institute, Ferry Lane, Kew, Surrey, TW9 3AS, England, under the provisions of the Budapest Treaty on the International Recognition of the Deposit of Micro-organisms for Patent Purposes.

* * * * *

Fig. 4.7.

You should begin by explaining the purpose for which the research has been done, especially if this has been to solve a particular technological problem. You should then identify and discuss prior published work on the subject with a view to explaining whether other effective solutions of the problem already exist or whether previous attempts at solving it have not fully succeeded. You then state in general terms the nature of your discovery or invention and how it achieves its objective. This must be followed by one or more detailed examples of the process or product or a drawing of the apparatus which will enable a person of ordinary skill in your particular field to carry out the invention in a practical way and achieve useful results.

The parts of the specification referred to above together make up the description of the invention which is addressed to the skilled person. In patent jargon he is spoken of as 'a person skilled in the art' and you will hear this expression used quite frequently in discussion or argument. The final part of the specification has a more legal function because it defines the scope of protection being sought by the applicant. This section is referred to as the 'Claims' and we will need to discuss this very important part of the document in more detail later.

The US Patent and Trade Mark Office issue guidelines for the preferred layout and content of patent applications. The suggested arrangement and headings are as follows:

> Title of invention
> Cross-references to related patent applications
> Field of invention (or technical field)
> Description of related art (or background art)
> Summary of invention

Description of the drawings and/or
Description of preferred embodiments (specific examples)
Claims

The European Patent Convention (EPC) sets out the desired 'Content of the description' in Rule 27 as follows.

(1) The description shall:

    (a) first state the title of the invention as appearing in the request for the grant of a European patent;

    (b) specify the technical field to which the invention relates;

    (c) indicate the background art which, as far as known to the applicant, can be regarded as useful for understanding the invention, for drawing up the European search report and for the examination, and, preferably, cite the documents reflecting such art;

    (d) disclose the invention, as claimed, in such terms that the technical problem (even if not expressly stated as such) and its solution can be understood, and state any advantageous effects of the invention with reference to the background art;

    (e) briefly describe the figures in the drawings, if any;

    (f) describe in detail at least one way of carrying out the invention claimed using examples where appropriate and referring to the drawings, if any;

    (g) indicate explicitly, when it is not obvious from the description or nature of the invention, the way in which the invention is capable of exploitation in industry.

(2) The description shall be presented in the manner and order specified in paragraph (1), unless, because of the nature of the invention, a different manner or a different order would afford a better understanding and a more economic presentation.

7   Must there have been a problem which the invention solves?

Patent Offices are more comfortable with specifications written in the style of a problem/solution presentation because it gives them something concrete to assess for inventive step (see EPC Rule 27 1(d) above). Most inventions which are patented are indeed aimed at solving an existing industrial or other technological problem and the practice of writing specifications has therefore become stereotyped in this way to a considerable extent. However, for the invention which comes 'out of the blue' as a fundamentally new product or process the drafting style can be modified. Even here, however, if the product or process is a radically new departure in itself there will still be a tendency to present the invention as meeting an existing need of some kind.

8   **How much literature searching should I do first?**

Presumably your research work has been preceded by or accompanied
by a literature search. At some stage you will want to have made a
complete search before you publish your work or present it as an
invention. The Patent Office and perhaps eventually also a court of law
will have to ask whether what you have done was new or obvious to any
skilled person in the state of scientific knowledge at the date of your
application, and this will include the entire available literature and
general scientific knowledge relevant to your field of research. The
assumption is that any other skilled person concerned to find a solution
of the problem on which you have worked will have made a diligent
search of prior knowledge. This may be a rather idealised view of how
things are done in research laboratories but if the law makes these
assumptions it would be wise to anticipate the kind of objections that
may be raised as a consequence.

The desirability of proper searching of the entire literature including
the scientific journals and patent literature can be justified for a number
of reasons. If there is an 'anticipation' in the prior art and neither you
nor your professional adviser knows of this, a great deal of time, effort,
and expense will have been involved needlessly and no useful result will
be obtained. Even if the prior knowledge is not a complete anticipation
of your work but is nevertheless pertinent to it under the aspects of
novelty and inventiveness, it could still vitally affect the way your
invention must be presented in order to be distinguishable from the
prior art. The specification can be amended after it has been filed at the
Patent Office but there are restrictions upon the applicant's freedom to
change what he has said and it may therefore prove rather difficult to
find your way through a minefield of prior publications of which you
were not previously aware or perhaps had ignored. This will be discussed
in more detail later when dealing with questions about novelty and
inventiveness as they arise in argument with the Patent Office.

Another important reason for a good early search is that the law of
the United States of America, and to some extent the laws of other
countries too, now require inventors and any other persons connected
with patent applications to bring everything to light which is relevant to
the question of patentability over the prior art. The applicant for
protection cannot place the entire burden of this assessment on the
shoulders of the Patent Office. An inventor is in conscience bound to
reveal all facts even those which may make his case more difficult if he is
to avoid any charge of fraud or deception in the process of obtaining
patent rights.

One of the Rules of Practice of the US Patent and Trade Mark Office (Rule 1.56) imposes the duty of candour and good faith on the inventor, attorney, or any other individual involved in the preparation and prosecution of a US patent application. These have a duty to disclose information material to the examination of the application. Accordingly Rules 1.97 and 1.98 encourage the filing of an 'Information Disclosure Statement' with or shortly after the filing of the application. This should list and be accompanied by copies of all patents, publications, and any other information which may be relevant background to the examination of the application. A concise statement of relevance is also required. Updating of this statement is desirable during prosecution of the application.

The main practical purpose of knowing in advance the prior art likely to be found in the official search, and also that which is not so easily discoverable, is that this is essential to the proper drafting of the patent claims defining the scope of protection.

9   What is meant by patent claims?

A patent claim is a verbal formula defining an invention. It is a definition of the new item of technology to which your work has given rise. It therefore recites in the most general way possible the new process, product, apparatus, or other subject matter in terms of its essential steps, structure, or component elements. A patent claim has nothing to do with a statement of the advantages of an invention over prior knowledge. In some cases the benefits or advantages that flow from the invention can be usefully mentioned in the claim e.g. in a clause saying 'whereby such and such a result is obtained' and this may be necessary or helpful in distinguishing the invention from prior art. However, functional clauses of this kind must be additional to the main structure or body of the claim language.

The function of the claim is not to tell the reader how to carry out the invention (the descriptive part of the specification does that) but is to define the scope of the legal protection and this therefore is a matter for professional draftsmen of patent specifications rather than the inventor. It is nevertheless important for an inventor to be able to look critically at patent claims from an informed point of view. It is conventional for a claim to be worded as a single sentence. It is also usual to have not only one claim but many claims differing from one another in scope and sometimes even in the terminology used where this is appropriate.

10   If the claims are so important, surely one ought to try to capture the underlying principle of the invention?

Yes and one always does subject to certain constraints. The underlying principle cannot be claimed in purely conceptual terms because a purely intellectual statement will not be recognised as an acceptable category of patentable invention. In a patent one is concerned with practical applications of the underlying principle in an economic context and that leads straight into the definition of processes and products. A claim such as 'utilising the principle of capillary action for delivering ink in a writing or drawing instrument' might be considered too indefinite for patent purposes (although it is a rather neat way of expressing the invention of the ball-point pen!). There is certainly room for more imagination in claim drafting but the regular established forms of claim are hard to displace.

11   How much can I cover in a single patent?

Normally one tries to cover as much as possible in one patent in order to obtain maximum value for money. The guiding principle, however, is that a patent covers a single invention. It is nevertheless possible in a single patent to cover subject matter linked by a common inventive concept and this is decided by examining the wording of the claims. This question is usually decided on formal Patent Office grounds such as whether the various claims cover subject matter in the same classification involving the same field of prior art search. An attempt to cover multiple inventions in one application will be noticed early in the process of examination and a formal objection will be raised. If one tries to be too ambitious to cover a wide ground over which the data are very thinly spread, the result may be unsatisfactory all round. It is a matter of judgement whether some aspects of the work should be reserved for separate patent applications filed at a later time when the development has been taken further so that they are well supported by data.

12   How much data must be provided for a sufficient patent disclosure?

The answer to Question 6 outlined the structure of the specification but more needs to be said. The basic idea of patent protection can be expressed as a bargain in which the parties both give to and receive from one another. The inventor teaches the skilled worker something new and gives the necessary information to enable this teaching to be put into practice. The European Patent Convention specifies that an application

> *'must disclose the invention in a manner sufficiently clear and complete for it to be carried out by a person skilled in the art' (Article 83).*

The corresponding section of United States patent law (Section 112) includes the following sentence:

> *'The specification shall contain a written description of the invention, and of the manner and process of making and using it, in such full, clear, concise, and exact terms as to enable any person skilled in the art to which it pertains, or with which it is most nearly connected, to make and use the same, and shall set forth the best mode contemplated by the inventor of carrying out his invention.'*

The concept of sufficiency of disclosure is universal in patent law and there is a fairly general consensus on it for non-biological inventions. In the biological field there is more diversity as to how to meet the sufficiency requirement as will be discussed in a later chapter.

Courts have in the past looked at this matter rather like a contract according to which the inventor's teaching is treated as the 'consideration' which must not fail if the contract is to be valid. The amount of information and guidance the inventor must give in the specification is therefore related to the extent of the legal protection requested, i.e. the scope of the claims. If for example a claim is presented which defines a product in very broad terms justice can be seen to be done only if the information given is commensurate with this claim scope. In chemistry this means that a claim to a large group of chemical compounds must be supported by practical detailed examples of the preparation or use of a reasonable number of representative specific compounds. Similarly in microbiology where the claim is not limited to individual strains of micro-organism or virus it will also be necessary to demonstrate by actual examples that the property or useful effect can be achieved across the range claimed. In fact the burden is greater in the case of living matter than for inanimate compounds. The UK Patent Office has rejected a claim to an alleged new species of micro-organism (exemplified by only one deposited strain) on the grounds that claims for novel micro-organisms must be confined to what has actually been discovered and cannot benefit from the degree of predictive generalisation normally acceptable for chemical inventions. (This problem will be discussed in more detail later with reference to patents for micro-organisms.) Similarly for process technology where it is asserted that the process may be carried out in a wide variety of alternative ways or steps it will be difficult to obtain wide cover if the working examples are confined to one particular set of the possible variables. If the Examiner objects that the supporting examples are too restrictive in relation to the scope of the claim it might be an effective answer to say that the examples actually given make it easy for the skilled worker to proceed by the alternative routes or steps which have been indicated in the specification, i.e. the reader does not have to exercise ingenuity in making the extrapolation. In some cases this argument might not be a reasonable one and the Examiner will reject it.

13   Presumably the Examples given in the patent specification must be a record of work done?

For inventions in the natural sciences this is usually the case but exceptions are possible. In answering Question 3 it was pointed out that inventions in certain branches of engineering are less demanding in this respect as compared with those in chemistry and microbiology. For the latter the specific worked patent Examples will correspond to the 'Materials and Methods' section of a scientific paper in which the experiments described have actually been performed by the author. However the function of a patent specification is to teach the skilled person how to carry out a process or make a new product and there is no reason in principle why an inventor should not include some 'prophetic' Examples together with those written around actual experiments.

It is up to the inventor to decide whether it is safe to extrapolate from actual results in order to instruct the skilled worker how the invention *could* be applied, say, to the preparation of specific products related to those which have been made by the inventor. There is clearly an element of risk in any extrapolation of this kind and many research workers are reluctant to take it for practical and even ethical reasons. However, where a broad patent claim is necessary, patent practice unfortunately demands that the inventor do something to counter the objection that an Examiner will raise if in his view the claim is not supported by the description. We have seen that it is futile to wait until the objection has been made before supplying additional data and therefore the patent agent will press the inventor to prepare the ground well in advance. In the more generally descriptive parts of a specification almost any patent will contain promises and will be predictive about the scope of application of an invention. Therefore the element of risk is always present because if these predictions are not borne out the patent will very likely be invalid on the ground of misleading and insufficient disclosure. Adding a few supportive and judiciously worded Examples of the kind contemplated can be justified on occasion but should preferably not be written in the past tense.

'Prophetic Examples' have been commented on by the United States Court of Appeals for the Federal Circuit in connection with the case of Atlas Powder v Du Pont over US Patent 3,447,978. The Court said: 'Du Pont contends that, because the '978 examples are "merely prophetic", they do not aid one skilled in the art in making the invention. Because they are prophetic, argues Du Pont, there can be no guarantee that the examples would actually work. Use of prophetic examples, however, does not automatically make a patent non-enabling. The burden is on one challenging validity to show by clear and convincing evidence that the prophetic examples together with other parts of the specification are not enabling. Du Pont did not meet that burden here. To the contrary, the District Court found that the "prophetic" examples of the specification were based on actual experiments that were slightly modified in the patent to reflect what the inventor believed to be optimum, and hence, they would be helpful in enabling someone to make the invention. Indeed, the District Court found that Du Pont's own researchers had little difficulty in making satisfactory emulsions with the emulsifying agents, salts, and fuels listed in the '978 patent.'

14   **I may not want to tell others everything about my invention. What will be the effect of keeping something back?**

You cannot have it both ways. If you leave out some essential item of information such that a person of ordinary skill in your field cannot obtain a useful result comparable with what you have asserted in the specification then the patent will be invalid. A skilled person is expected to supplement the written description you have given from the stock of knowledge he can be assumed to possess. But if for some reason he cannot reproduce anything like the results you have claimed and cannot readily see where he might be going wrong the inventor has not fulfilled his side of the bargain. Also in the quotation from United States patent law given in answer to Question 12 the need for the inventor to disclose the best mode known to him of carrying out his invention is obligatory if the patent is to be sustained. This rules out any idea of holding back any important information. The inventor will need to discuss this question fairly thoroughly with his professional adviser because one might want to draw a line between information that must be included in the specification and information which is more in the nature of know-how which is not amenable to written description in a practically convenient way.

15   **Must I include in the specification details of materials and methods if these are already in the scientific or patent literature?**

A certain amount of cross-reference to published work is acceptable and convenient. For example the composition of certain well known culture media can be dealt with by mentioning the appropriate scientific reference. If this kind of shorthand is overdone, however, it will convey the impression that too much of what is supposed to be the novel teaching of the inventor is already in the public domain. Even if the relevant information can be taken from published work it is better to transport it in your own words into the specification so that the latter is as self-contained as possible. The Examiner will expect this to be done so that he can judge the sufficiency of the disclosure on the text in front of him.

Cross-reference to prior work cannot be relied on as a substitute for actually doing the necessary experimental work yourself to apply published methods to your own specific invention.

16   **Who is the 'inventor' for the purposes of patent law?**

According to the legal meaning the inventor is the actual deviser of what is being claimed. Frequently there may be more than one inventor because it has taken two or more persons to arrive at the conception or realisation of the final process or product. This does not mean that every single person who has worked on the research project must be named as a co-inventor. Entities should not be multiplied unnecessarily. The naming of inventors must be restricted to those who have made key contributions either in the research strategy or in the actual experimental discoveries. It is incorrect to include those who have merely carried out experiments under complete direction from others.

17   **How does one decide who are the 'inventors'?**

This is a matter of judgment primarily for your professional adviser who will know of the legal decisions (admittedly rather few) affecting this question. Your adviser will therefore guide you in this but he has to be told the important facts about the initial devising of the research topic, the way the results have unfolded, and the people who have made key contributions along the way.

18   **How important is the question of inventorship?**

It is important for a number of reasons. The legal rights in an invention are originally with the inventors but vest finally with whoever is entitled to them. This entitlement may remain with the inventors or it may not. The most common situation is that an inventor holds his inventive rights in trust for his employer or some other funding body either because the law says so or because a contract has been previously made which covers the question of ownership. The question of inventorship must therefore be settled before the related question of ownership can be answered. If this question is approached in a careless way the resulting patent could be invalid. Apart from these practical reasons it is only right to give public recognition of the true origin of an invention.

19   **Does it really matter who the inventors are if there is a common owner of the rights anyway?**

Even though all the inventors may be bound to assign their rights to a common owner e.g. an industrial employer it is still necessary to be accurate over inventorship. Should inventorship be challenged for any reason it is important to be able to justify the original naming of the inventors and to show that this has been carried out responsibly. In the USA patent applications are filed in the names of inventors as applicants even though an assignment of their rights to their corporation or some other party is in existence. This gives the inventors a formal status which merits a truly professional approach to the legal question.

20   **It is often difficult to recall from whom the particular ideas or key suggestions originated. Is it not safer to name every member of the team?**

It may indeed be difficult to disentangle individual contributions. Apart from that there may be a temptation to fudge the issue because it is too painful to exclude anyone and because it involves some tedious hair-splitting. You must simply make a sincere attempt to approach a legal question in a legal way. The main burden of this investigation lies upon the professional adviser whose duty it is to ask the appropriate questions which should bring out the important points. It is useful to record reasons why certain members of the team are considered to have made inventive contributions whereas others have not. These contributions do not have to be of equal merit and if one is dealing with a team of objective and dispassionate co-workers they might even agree on an apportionment of merit which may be relevant to the sharing of ultimate benefit.

21   **Among a group of collaborators there may be some who perhaps do not qualify legally as co-inventors but who have played an important part in the success of the work. How does the law deal with such a situation?**

The law itself does not deal with this situation. It is nevertheless a common occurrence and the parties concerned should themselves seek an equitable solution.

22   **If inventorship is wrongly assessed can this be cured later?**

If discovered in time an error in the inventorship can be corrected but this usually involves swearing affidavits or making formal declarations explaining the error and how it arose. That process can be tedious and embarrassing for all concerned. The correction of a 'misjoinder' of inventors in United States patent practice is a field in which there is much experience and one to which much importance is attached. In USA the inventors are the actual applicants for the patent even though they may have assigned their rights to a corporation or other party. The party to which the rights have been assigned is the 'assignee' and his rights are usually recorded in the Patent Office as legal owner even though the patent is applied for and nominally granted to the inventors.

23   **After starting the patenting process on the lines advocated above what can be done if the research does not progress (a) fast enough or (b) in accordance with the initial ideas?**

This question presupposes that the inventor has not held back from patenting until the invention has been thoroughly researched and the data are extensive and confirmed. This is indeed the normal case. In a competitive environment patenting has often to be started while research is still on-going and new results are continually modifying or correcting early ideas. The question deals with both the pace of research and the direction of research; these are distinct items although one solution may be common to both. If problems are met under either heading the simplest solution is to scrap the first attempt and to start afresh. Some of the implications of a stop and re-start policy need to be understood.

(a)   Speed of research

When a patent application is filed it establishes a priority right as of the date of filing for whatever it discloses. Therefore provided the research is soundly based and well described in the specification the priority date of the first filing can be very important in relation to competitive research workers and publications which appear after the application has been filed. Inevitably however part of the original specification may be speculative and written in the optimistic belief that confirmatory results will soon flow from the laboratory bench. In some countries there is a facility for treating the first filing as a record of priority only i.e. without pursuing it through to the final grant of a patent. Instead, the first filing can be superseded by a second application filed within one year of the first which can update and develop the original disclosure and can claim a relationship with the first filing. That is, the second application will claim the priority date of the first filing for whatever is disclosed in the latter and is reproduced in the second application. Because of this important aspect of patent practice in some countries a certain amount of forward thinking can be included in the first application and substantiated in more detail in the second application whilst at the same time probably benefiting from the earlier date for priority purposes. Moreover this ability to interconnect two applications filed within one year of each other has even greater value and importance in relation to foreign patenting under the International Convention which has been mentioned briefly in the answer to Question 6 of Chapter 3. This, the Paris Convention, allows foreign patent applications to be accorded the priority date of the first application in a contracting state (a Convention country) provided the foreign application is filed within one year of the priority application. It goes without saying that the subject matter of the foreign application must be disclosed in the priority application.

In view of the fact that patent applications are not immediately published but remain secret within the Patent Office it will be appreciated that if the experimental development of the invention within the year following the first filing is slower than expected, with the result that one is not in a position to file an effective second application within the Convention year, it is possible to abandon the first application and to start the process over again with a new time-table. This is known as 'abandon and refile' tactics and is often resorted to by applicants with limited research funds and other resources. Of course it involves the sacrifice of the original priority date and a fall-back to a later priority date (the application date of the refiled application).

It follows that abandon and refile tactics can generally only be used where the applicant or inventor has not published details of the invention after the first filing date because, in relation to the later filing date, the inventor's own disclosure will have become part of the prior art except where a grace period can be utilised. This reservation has also to be made as regards open exploitation of an invention after the first filing date which amounts either to a prior publication or a prior use of the invention.

(b)   The direction of research

We are concerned here not with a failure, through lack of time, to substantiate the promises made in the original application but a situation in which further research has shown that the original specification is in need of substantial revision. Where significant changes have to be made in the way the invention is formulated there may be little alternative than to start afresh. It all depends on the degree of divergence from the original statement of ideas and results. So long as a significant part of the original specification is still a valid way of describing the invention it would be better to adhere to the original deadline for taking appropriate action. It is a matter of professional judgement as to how much can be salvaged from the original application. A fresh start will usually be preferable in these circumstances; some priority will have been lost but against this there is the advantage of starting afresh with a more accurate and well supported presentation of the invention. Of course, the possibility of intervening publication by the inventor himself or by some third party must be taken into account.

It would be appropriate to conclude this answer with a summary of patent procedure and timescales which will reinforce the points made in answer to this question.

Summary of patent procedure

The time-scale of patent procedure is illustrated in Figure 4.8. The general plan of international patenting procedure is shown giving some idea of the stages and the typical times involved before the results are known.

An application for patent protection is normally first made in the country of residence or place of business of the applicant. This establishes a so-called priority date which will be recognised in most of the other countries of the world under the provisions of an international convention known as the Paris Convention. In practice this means that the major expense of a foreign patenting programme can be postponed until towards the end of one year after the initial filing date in the home country. For this purpose an application for a European (regional) patent is on the same footing as national applications in other countries filed under the Paris Convention. The value of this one-year interim period, both to industry and to other organisations which have the problem of assessing the potential industrial importance of new research results, is considerable. The other major advantage given by the Paris Convention is that the inventor can publish details of his invention at any time after his priority date without detriment to his patent prospects. The only provisos here are that the invention is clearly

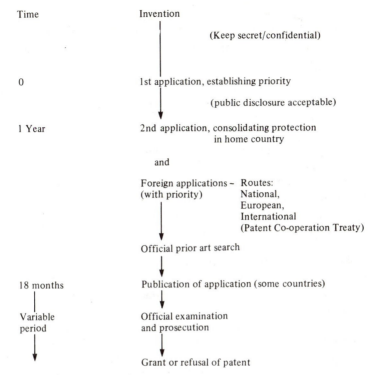

Fig. 4.8. Patenting procedure

defined and well supported by data in the specification filed with the first application and that the foreign applications are filed no later than one year after the first application.

The need for secrecy or strict confidentiality in the period between making an invention and filing for patent protection has already been strongly emphasised. After the first filing, public disclosure is acceptable so long as the effective foundation for protection has been laid. At the one-year stage, at which foreign cover may be sought, the cost element becomes a major consideration and must be carefully considered well before the deadline arrives. The routes to foreign protection will be explained later. The next significant stage involves the official reaction to the application(s) first in the form of a prior art search following which publication of the application will occur in some countries. Thus in European countries the search of prior art and the subsequent examination for patentability are separate stages of procedure. If the applicant wishes to persevere after seeing the search results the examination and prosecution stage will then commence and continue until a conclusion is reached. In USA, Canada and Japan, however, search and examination are carried out as a single operation.

24   **In contrast to the previous question, suppose the research is continually developing and generating modifications and new findings in quick succession. How can these be accommodated in the patent?**

When an application is filed, you have 'started the clock' and most of what has to follow will be governed by deadlines prescribed by law. This applies unless you abandon and refile and thereby re-start the clock. Consequently there is a cut-off date beyond which new developments cannot be incorporated into the one application.

In the one-year period between the first filing and the filing of the consolidating application, and foreign applications under the Paris Convention, everything can be accommodated. This is done by filing additional applications so that towards the end of the priority year (or Convention year, as it is also called) you will have a series of applications from which a single omnibus application can be put together by the scissors and paste method. Alternatively you may have to distribute the subject matter among two or more applications, rather than one omnibus, because separate inventive concepts have emerged which require separate treatment.

After the consolidation mentioned above has taken place, new data arising must be dealt with by subsequent patent applications. In the law of most countries, so long as the first or consolidated application has not yet been published, the application will not be counted as prior art relevant to the inventiveness of any new application. Once the original invention has been published, however, the new invention must be patentably distinguished from it and the new application is not legally inter-related with the first.

US patent practice is unique in allowing the relationship between the first and subsequent applications to be extended by means of so-called continuation and continuation-in-part applications. Continuation applications do not and cannot include new data and are simply a means of prolonging the process of prosecution of the original invention disclosure by refiling the original specification as a new application entitled to the priority date of the earlier one. Continuation-in-part applications usually reproduce most if not all of the original specification but they add new matter which is entitled only to its own filing date for purposes of assessing priority. Seemingly, continuation-in-part practice appears ideally suited to the constantly developing research project but it can only be used safely under proper professional advice. The subtleties cannot be fully explained here and one simply has to depend for guidance on the US attorney, who ought to be kept fully informed of research strategy and progress as it develops or preferably before!

25 How are prosecution and examination of the application carried out?

This is done chiefly by correspondence between the Patent Office and the applicant's agent, or the applicant himself if he chooses to apply without professional help. The Examiner will issue an official letter or official 'action', as it is so called, in which objections will be raised against the claims or over the way the invention has been described in the specification. The most common objection is that the claims presented are not allowable in view of the prior art, which must be specified by the Examiner. A period or 'term' for response will be set giving a few months for the applicant to make an effective reply which either rebuts the Examiner's arguments or amends the scope of the claims so that they are distinguished from the prior art and define an invention which is patentable over it. Usually extensions of time for response are available upon payment of an extra official fee so that the applicant may have as much as four or even six months in which to re-evaluate his position and produce the necessary counter-arguments and information required in support of these. This period can turn out to be rather short, especially if more experimental work is necessary to produce evidence to justify the applicant's standpoint. The applicant's response will be considered by the Examiner and a further official action issued if necessary, whereupon the process will be repeated until agreement is reached. Personal interview with the Examiner is also possible and will often short-cut the correspondence. The applicant can appeal against an adverse decision of the Examiner. It is not uncommon, therefore, for prosecution to continue for two or three years or more.

5 Meeting requirements: the cornerstones of patent law

Previous chapters have made it clear that obtaining patent protection depends on meeting certain requirements or criteria of patentability in the process known as prosecuting the patent application. The four most important requirements may be likened to cornerstones or foundations upon which the whole elaborate superstructure rests. Three of these concern the invention itself, namely, it must have (1) novelty, (2) inventiveness and (3) practical utility or industrial applicability while the other (4) concerns the specification; this must be adequate in content to enable those of ordinary skill and experience in the field to follow the directions and obtain the promised results. The application of these criteria in practice often involves legal subtleties, as will be described later, but they may be simply summarised in the following recapitulation of points discussed in previous chapters.

Novelty

This condition requires that the invention must not already be available to others by any kind of public disclosure or use before the date of filing of the patent application. Although the rule is commonly expressed in terms of 'publication' it is important to note that this includes all forms of public disclosure and is not limited to literature publication. It covers all forms of publication, disclosure and use previous to the patent application, even those made by or due to the inventor himself. All such prior knowledge etc. is known as the 'state of the art' or 'prior art'. Prior experimental use which occurs within the privacy of the research laboratory is not part of the state of the art so long as the details remain as private or restricted information. A disclosure by an inventor can sometimes be confidential, as distinct from public, and this does not destroy novelty. This outline of the novelty rules applies to most countries but the United States, Canada, Japan and a few others are exceptions in allowing grace periods for filing patent applications in their respective countries after publication or use by the inventor.

Inventiveness

The invention must not be 'obvious' to the ordinary skilled worker over the state of the art, i.e. it must not follow plainly or logically from what is already known. Research workers who write literature publications which present their work as a natural logical scientific development from prior published papers make it difficult for themselves to argue that it has inventive character.

Utility or industrial application

Utility is a crucial concept in US patent law but is not limited to industrial utility and any other sort of practical utility can suffice. In European law an invention must be capable of industrial application.

Adequate disclosure

The description of the invention must be such as to permit repetition of the work by a person of normal skill. This criterion has led to special problems with biological inventions in that it is often difficult or even impossible to define living organisms or their products with sufficient precision to ensure reproducibility.

The statements made above are precise and fairly clear-cut but invariably stimulate questions of the following kind.

1 **What exactly is meant by 'new'? Does it mean something which is fundamentally new or will a new application of a known technique be patentable?**

This question must be answered in relation to what is defined in the patent claims. To be new the process, product, or apparatus which is defined in the precise terms of the claims must be something which cannot be found in the prior art. The various components of the claim can therefore be considered as a check list to be ticked off against any particular prior document or prior use which is considered to be relevant. Moreover to defeat a claim on the ground of lack of novelty the whole of what is claimed must have been described in the particular document or must have been used in the particular prior user. In the majority of cases the invention, considered in this way, will not be totally new in every one of its component parts. The invention may be the novel application of known things. In the chemical or microbiological patent literature for example many of the new products patented will be prepared by a combination of conventional synthetic or fermentation reactions which happen not to have been combined before to convert a particular starting material into a particular new product. So long as the end result is not already anticipated by explicit reference in the prior art the patent law does not insist on totally new reactions and reaction mechanisms.

2   **So you could patent a combination of known steps or bits of apparatus so long as the combination could not be found described in a prior document or in any other form of prior art?**

Yes. Every step of a process and every individual part of an apparatus can be suggested, described or otherwise known in the prior art and yet the combination may be novel. The same can be said for compositions containing various substances. The process or apparatus therefore passes the novelty hurdle and progresses to the next one at which the question will be whether a particular combination is hinted at or implied in the prior art. This next hurdle is the question of inventive step which will be discussed below.

3   **Can novelty reside in the intended purpose of the process or product?**

In considering a claim for a product it is the thing itself that must be new. Where the product is a substance the claim will be to the substance as such and therefore if a substance of the same composition or identity is already disclosed in the literature or other prior art it does not have absolute novelty *per se*.

4   **In the circumstances of the previous question can you not patent a product 'for use in' a specific new application?**

It is possible to use the 'product for use' type of claim in European patent law where the product, considered solely as an entity in itself, is not new but where it has been discovered for the first time to have a biological utility. The classical example of this would be a chemical compound described in the chemical literature but without reference to any biological activity. In such a case a 'product X for use in the treatment of disease Y' or a similar type of claim involving a therapeutic or prophylactic use would be acceptable. This is straightforward as regards product claims. As regards process claims for a new application of an otherwise known process it is usually much easier to incorporate procedural novelty into the words of the claim.

The usual case is where product X is biologically active. However, this type of claim can also be used where X is not itself active but is useful in association with another material which is active, as in UK Patent 2,126,081 which claims

> *'a polymer which is permselective with respect to fluoride ions and which comprises both hydrophobic groups and backbone phosphate groups, for use in dental prophylaxis or therapy'.*

In the USA and most other countries the 'product for use' claim is not formally available and the claim will have to be expressed in terms of a formulation of the active product appropriate to the biological use. Method of use claims are also available in the USA.

5   Suppose the product is already known for one biological application but a different biological utility is discovered?

In the European Patent Office this point has been specifically decided at high level and patent protection can be obtained for the so-called second indication. In this situation the 'product for use' claim is not allowed. The form of claim permitted is known as a 'purpose-limited process of manufacture claim' and it will usually be expressed in the form of 'use of product X for the manufacture of a medicament for the treatment of disease Y'.

> *The particular case decided by the Appeal Board of the European Patent Office concerned the drug nimodipin which had been first patented as a product useful in the treatment of cardiac conditions but not actively pursued for this purpose. The drug was subsequently found to increase cerebral blood flow and therefore to be useful for the treatment of other medical conditions, e.g. senility. Promotion of nimodipin for this use involved clinical trials and other costly development work by its proprietor, the German company Bayer ag, which justified making it a test case for patent protection for the second medical indication. The EPO decision was also followed in the UK and elsewhere and in subsequent cases involving a similar principle.*

6   Can you overcome the effect of a prior document by questioning its credibility?

The Examiner is entitled to draw attention to any prior document that in his view discloses your invention or something very close to it. The fact that this earlier reported work may not have been properly carried out scientifically is irrelevant to the question of novelty so long as the disclosure itself covers what you are claiming. For example the earlier paper may not have supplied sufficient evidence to justify its conclusions or for other reasons may not have proved its own case but the Examiner is not concerned with that issue. The Examiner can cite science fiction if the disclosure is at all relevant to your invention. Furthermore the earlier work may well have had a different objective and may only incidentally or accidentally touch on what is relevant to the subject matter you are now presenting as new and inventive. The test is always how the skilled person, working on the same problem as yourself, would have read and interpreted the prior disclosure. It is often possible to dismiss a cited prior publication on the ground that the work was so badly done that no research worker of any standing would take much notice of it. However this is only possible when the inventiveness, as distinct from the novelty, of your work is being questioned. If the previous paper discloses the subject matter of your claims as drafted then the lack of novelty objection is a serious one.

Sometimes a prior document is cited which discloses something which will not work as stated or will not work at all. Some patent specifications come into this category. Again the argument that the prior teaching is inoperative can be deployed effectively when one requires to establish an inventive step but is much more difficult to sustain if the various parts of your patent claim can all be found together in the cited specification or other prior document. If you use the inoperativeness argument the Examiner may respond that your own claim must be distinguished from the prior art by limiting it to the combination of conditions or other features which are necessary to make the process or product work and which are not disclosed in the prior art.

7   **It would be helpful to summarise what has been said about novelty and to give practical examples.**

Dealing first with the question of product claims we will assume that the invention is a product of a chemical or microbiological process or is a living organism.

(a)   The product is new

The product is a new synthetic or biosynthetic substance or a hitherto unknown natural product or organism isolated for the first time. A product patent is obtainable in these circumstances containing a claim to the substance or organism *per se.* The product must be defined by chemical structure or by some other acceptable method. To support a claim of this kind the specification will typically include details of the preparation or isolation of the substance or organism. There must also be some statement of the properties of the product and preferably an appropriate demonstration of these properties, e.g. *in vitro* or *in vivo.*

(b)   The product is old

In patent jargon a product is 'old' if it has already been described in the literature or used in the prior art, even for a different purpose. Assuming no biological properties have been attributed to the known substance it will be possible to obtain 'product for use' claims in some countries, and composition claims or unit dosage formulation claims in others. Method of use claims, i.e. covering the treatment of a human or animal, will be refused in most countries apart from USA but this will not be serious so long as commercially valuable product or composition claims can be obtained.

As under (a) it will be necessary to provide supporting disclosure for the statement of biological properties.

(c)   The product is known for a different biological utility

Here the availability of product or composition claims depends mainly on whether the product has to be formulated in a special way for the new biological use (a different method of administering the product may be necessary). Claims to a method of treatment of a human or animal using the product will be refused in most countries if the object of treatment is essentially medical (therapeutic or prophylactic). Claims to methods of treatment for an economic purpose, e.g. increasing the weight of animals or the ratio of lean to fat, are acceptable. In the USA methods of treatment of all kinds can be obtained , i.e. medical as well as economic. As before, appropriate biological demonstration must be provided. Where the claims are method of treatment claims there must be a description of the actual method claimed with particular details of such treatment. With product claims it is often possible to extrapolate from experimental trials in the mouse, rat, etc., but where the claim is to a method of treatment the exemplification must be more direct.

8   **How is the new use of a known material or a known apparatus treated from the point of view of novelty?**

A material, device, or apparatus which is already known for one purpose cannot be patented just because a new use or application has been discovered or is proposed for it. What may be patentable is the new use or method or process involved and the claim may be expressed in any of these ways. However if the new use requires some modification of the known material etc. this may be sufficient to introduce bare novelty in what is claimed. This is a common situation where in order to work properly in a new use an apparatus for example may need one additional item or one component different from the prior form of the equipment. A particular physical form of an otherwise known material, e.g. a particle size distribution, may also be sufficient to comply with the novelty requirement. Small differences may be critical to success in the new use. New uses of this general type often raise questions of inventive step rather than of novelty and therefore present more difficulty in patent law (see below).

9   **In considering novelty is it necessary to take into account earlier patent applications which are still pending?**

In a great many countries earlier patent applications are considered to be part of the state of the art against later applications filed in the same legal jurisdiction. In European patent law prior EPC applications are citable as far as novelty is concerned but are disregarded for the purposes of considering inventiveness. To be citable it is necessary for the earlier patent application eventually to proceed to publication; if this does not take place because the application is abandoned for any reason before publication it is disregarded for all purposes. The entire disclosure of the earlier application ('whole contents') is taken into consideration for this purpose irrespective of whether there is any conflict between the claims of the earlier and later applications.

In US patent law earlier applications are also prior art so long as they result in granted patents. On grant of a patent the earlier application is treated as prior art from its *application* date. Moreover, unlike in the European parallel, this applies for the purposes of determining both the novelty and the inventiveness of the later applicant's invention.

The consequence of this is that an element of uncertainty in searching the prior art must always persist as regards the more recent years of the search. Under the European system this is less serious because European applications are published whilst they are still applications whereas US patent applications are not published so long as their application status remains.

10   **Inventiveness must be difficult to judge and impossible to quantify. How does patent law cope with this problem?**

Patent law postulates the existence of the quality of inventiveness and the idea of an inventive step forward from the prior art. Unlike in the case of novelty, however, where the legal definition is precise, the written law does not attempt to define the criteria of inventiveness except to say that something involves an inventive step if it is not *obvious* to the skilled person in the light of the state of the art. According to US patent law even though the alleged invention is not identically disclosed in the prior art a patent may not be obtained

> 'if the difference between the subject matter sought to be patented and the prior art are such that the subject matter as a

whole would have been obvious at the time the invention was made to a person having ordinary skill in the art to which said subject matter pertains.'

The US Patent Office Examiner is allowed to assert that the subject matter of the patent application before him is obvious to those skilled in the art and he is not obliged to supply an argument that supports his assertion. The burden is placed upon the applicant to show why such a criticism is unjustified.

A European Patent Office Examiner is entitled to make the same objection of lack of inventive step and in this he has to follow the guidelines established by the European Patent Office. The relevant guideline interprets the term 'obvious' in the following way:

> 'The term 'obvious' means that which does not go beyond the normal progress of technology but merely follows plainly or logically from the prior art, i.e. something which does not involve the exercise of any skill or ability beyond that to be expected of the person skilled in the art.'

The guideline then gives a number of examples with suggested answers as to whether a conclusion of obviousness or non-obviousness would follow. To avoid discouraging the inventor the guideline concludes with the following statement:

> 'It should be remembered that an invention which at first sight appears obvious might in fact involve an inventive step. Once a new idea has been formulated it can often be shown theoretically how it might be arrived at, starting from something known, by a series of apparently easy steps. The examiner should be wary of *ex post facto* analysis of this kind. He should always bear in mind that the documents produced in the search have, of necessity, been obtained with foreknowledge of what matter constitutes the alleged invention. In all cases he should attempt to visualise the overall state of the art confronting the skilled man before the applicant's contribution and he should seek to make a "real life" assessment of this and other relevant factors. He should take into account all that is known concerning the background of the invention and give fair weight to relevant arguments or evidence submitted by the applicant. If, for example, an invention is shown to be of considerable technical value, and particularly if it provides a technical advantage which is new and surprising, and this can convincingly be related to one or more of the features included in the claim defining the invention, the examiner should be hesitant in pursuing an objection that such a claim lacks inventive step. The same applies where the invention solves a

technical problem which workers in the art have been
attempting to solve for a long time, or otherwise fulfils a long-
felt need. Commercial success alone is not to be regarded as
indicative of inventive step, but evidence of immediate
commercial success when coupled with evidence of a long-felt
want is of relevance provided the examiner is satisfied that the
success derives from the technical features of the invention and
not from other influences (e.g. selling techniques or
advertising).'

The European Patent Office has in these guidelines provided the best
help given so far by any official body to inventors and patent attorneys
in the difficult business of assessing patent prospects in the light of the
objections that might possibly be raised.

Ultimately the difficult business of coping with the practical
application of these principles is left to the courts and the patent
lawyers. These are helped by the evidence of expert witnesses who can
be brought in to assist in the evaluation. The expertise of these witnesses
is not usually in patent law but in the technical art to which the patent
relates.

11   **In considering inventiveness how do you assess the level of
knowledge possessed by the so-called person skilled in the art?**

The concept of a 'person of ordinary skill' or, as he is curiously described
in European parlance, the 'average expert' is one which patent law has
relied upon from early times. The ordinary skilled worker is the person
to whom a patent specification is supposed to be addressed in the
relevant field of technology. He is somewhere to be found in the
spectrum which contains Nobel Prize winners at one end and laboratory
technicians at the other. Therefore he is assumed to have an ordinary
level of skill and knowledge and cannot really be styled as 'expert' in the
usually accepted sense. However the knowledge available to this person
is at the same time assumed to be vast. He is supposed to be aware of or
to have ready access to the entire literature and totality of recorded
knowledge relevant to the field in which he works. He is also assumed
to have the ability to connect together separate items of knowledge from
the whole of space-time in so far as these have a bearing upon the
question of inventive step. He is a necessary part of the Patent Office
Examiner's argument when the Examiner wishes to deny the
inventiveness of what is being claimed in a patent application.

The Examiner will confidently assert that many things are obvious to
the skilled person by piecing together bits from different parts of the
literature and even from different technologies. In this respect the
patent law seems highly artificial to inventors who know that their

colleagues and counterparts in real life do not correspond at all well to such a concept. The real person of ordinary skill has only a limited amount of knowledge at the operative level of consciousness and usually has a rather narrower approach to the field he needs to search manually or by computer in order to arrive at an appreciation of prior work which is truly relevant to his own research.

The Examiner will often state that, as of the filing date of the patent application he is examining, it would have been obvious to the skilled person to do what is being claimed in view of prior reference A combined with prior reference B etc. or selected passages from each. This type of argument is one of theoretical speculation and there are occasions when it is justified in practice and many more when it is not. It is always easy after the event to find prior literature or other references which seem to make the subsequent invention obvious. This is the classic hindsight approach and is quite erroneous. Occasionally it is possible to show from work published by other research workers *after* the patent application date that real life experts did not in fact come to the conclusions that the Examiner considers were obvious at the relevant date. This is a powerful argument against obviousness which some courts are more ready to listen to than those Examiners who attribute omniscience to the hypothetical figure in their imagination. The EPO guideline on this subject mentioned above is a refreshingly helpful approach to this problem and it is hoped that Examiners will adhere to it in practice.

12   What is the difference between utility and industrial applicability?

The US patent law requires that an invention be useful and this stems from the origin of the patent system as promoting the 'useful arts'. There are other useful arts than those of the industrial sphere and the US law is therefore most liberal in this respect. Utility does have a practical connotation, however, as distinct from the theoretical. A method of solving a mathematical equation might not be patentable insofar as it depended solely on a series of mental steps. But a new method of filling a tooth would be patentable in the USA even though it has nothing to do with industry.

In Europe the test is that an invention must be 'susceptible of industrial application' and EPC Article 57 explains that this means capable of being 'made or used in any kind of industry, including agriculture'. This is developed further in the European Patent Office Guidelines which state that:

> 'Industry' should be understood in its broad sense as including any physical activity of "technical character", i.e. an activity

which belongs to the useful or practical arts as distinct from the aesthetic arts; it does not necessarily imply the use of a machine or the manufacture of an article and could cover e.g. a process for dispersing fog, or a process for converting energy from one form to another. Thus, Article 57 excludes from patentability very few "inventions" which are not already excluded by the list in Article 52, paragraph 2.'

The chief difference between European and United States law on this subject lies in the specific exclusion of certain types of method from patentability under the EPC. The European Patent Office guidelines explain this as follows:

'Methods for treatment of the human or animal body by surgery or therapy and diagnostic methods practised on the human or animal body shall not be regarded as inventions which are susceptible of industrial application. This provision shall not apply to products, in particular substances or compositions, for use in any of these methods. Patents may, however, be obtained for surgical, therapeutic or diagnostic instruments or apparatus for use in such methods. Also the manufacture of prostheses or artificial limbs, as well as taking measurements therefor on the human body, would be patentable, so that a method of manufacturing a prosthetic tooth which involves making a model of a patient's teeth in the mouth would not be excluded from patentability. Patents may also be obtained for new products for use in these methods of treatment or diagnosis, particularly substances or compositions.'

'It should be noted that Article 52, paragraph 4, excludes only treatment by surgery or therapy or diagnostic methods. It follows that other methods of treatment of live human beings or animals (e.g. treatment of a sheep in order to promote growth, to improve the quality of mutton or to increase the yield of wool) or other methods of measuring or recording characteristics of the human or animal body are patentable provided that (as would probably be the case) such methods are of a technical and not essentially biological character and provided that the methods are susceptible of industrial application. The latter proviso is particularly important in the case of human beings. A treatment or diagnostic method, to be excluded, must actually be carried out on the living human or animal body. A treatment of or diagnostic method practised on a dead human or animal body would therefore not be excluded from patentability by virtue of Article 52, paragraph 4. Treatment of body tissues or fluids after they have been removed from the human or animal body, or diagnostic methods applied thereon, are not excluded from patentability in so far as these tissues or fluids are not returned to the same body. Thus the treatment of blood for storage in a blood bank or diagnostic testing of blood samples is not excluded, whereas a treatment of blood by dialysis with the blood being returned to the same body would be excluded. Diagnostic methods comprise the carrying out of an investigation for medical purposes into the state of a human or animal body; so that a method of measuring the blood pressure of a body or a method of obtaining information regarding the internal state of a body by passing X-rays through the body would be excluded from patentability. A treatment by therapy implies the curing of a disease or malfunction of the body; prophylactic methods, e.g. immunisation, are considered to be therapeutic treatments and thus excluded. Surgery is not limited to healing treatments, being more indicative of the nature of the treatment; methods of cosmetic surgery are thus excluded from patentability.

Methods of testing generally should be regarded as inventions susceptible of industrial application and therefore patentable if the test is applicable to the improvement or control of a product, apparatus or process which is itself susceptible of industrial application. In particular, the utilisation of test animals for test purposes in industry, e.g. for testing industrial products (for example for ascertaining the absence of pyrogenetic or allergic effect) or phenomena (for example for determining water or air pollution) would be patentable.'

13   **Why does European patent law exclude the methods referred to above?**

The exclusion of the above methods of treatment from patentability in European law is said to be justified on ethical grounds. Patenting such methods is possible under US law and not perceived as an ethical problem or one which gives rise to any real difficulties between doctor and patient in that country. It is difficult to see why the European exclusion should cover animals as well as humans. Most treatments in animal health care are designed for practical reasons related to the principal economic purposes of rearing animals in the first place. Since it has been made clear that agriculture is an industry for the purposes of patent law there seems to be an internal contradiction in the law which ought to be removed.

14   What is meant by 'adequate disclosure' of an invention?

This topic has been partly covered in Chapter 4 in answer to Question 12 and later questions. It arises as part of preparing a patent application and is of vital importance to making a proper start on the patenting process. A defective disclosure usually cannot be cured after a patent application has been filed because the examiner will reject any attempt to add new matter into an application. The legal requirement is usually expressed as sufficiency of disclosure, enabling disclosure, reproducible teaching, or in similar terms.

As for the test for inventiveness discussed in answer to Question 11 the test of adequacy of disclosure is applied to the person skilled in the art. Theoretically the notional person skilled in the art should be the same for both criteria but it is better to err on the safe side and provide as much information as possible in a patent application to ensure that someone of ordinary skill will have no legitimate reason for failing to reproduce the work described.

The problem of enabling disclosure is particularly acute in the biological field and is best dealt with more fully in the next chapter.

15   What are the consequences of error in the patent description?

This depends so much on the context that to give too firm a general answer would be dangerous. Errors which are obvious on the face of the document can usually be corrected wherever the local practice allows for an application to amend the description voluntarily or where the correction can be made in the course of making other amendments to overcome official objections. An obvious inconsistency between various parts of the description can usually be put right when it is clear which of the conflicting statements or data is the wrong one.

In the generous practice of the European Patent Office it has been allowed in a chemical case to correct a wrong numerical value given for the quantity of catalyst used in one of the detailed Examples given in the specification. It was shown that the Example could not be faithfully repeated using the quantities of reagents and catalyst given but it was held that the skilled worker would realise the discrepancy and from observation of the reaction would easily see what corrective action to take.

6   Microbiological inventions

It is convenient to treat the subject matter of this chapter more formally and to depart from the direct question and answer method used until now.

The principles of patent law outlined in earlier chapters are of general application to inventions in all technologies. It is appropriate now to focus on the specific area of biotechnology inventions and the distinctive problems which are met in the patenting of these. In the written statutes of patent law it is not the practice to single out any particular technology for attention except where specific items are excluded from patentability, e.g. computer programs, plant and animal varieties, and methods of diagnosis and medical treatment all of which cannot be patented under European law. Patent law does not refer to 'biotechnology', a term not yet in common use when many of the more recent patent laws were written. The European Patent Convention refers to 'microbiological processes' or the 'products of microbiological processes' and these are referred to generally as 'microbiological inventions'. We can assume that a microbiological invention is one involving a micro-organism but patent law has so far shown no inclination to define the term micro-organism. This turns out to have been a wise intuition because it has allowed the practices worked out for inventions involving, say, bacteria and fungi to be extended pragmatically to other biological entities which replicate or can be made to replicate, e.g. plasmids, viruses and cell lines.

The general character of patent law has been shaped long before the advent of the new biotechnology and is designed to embrace a whole range of different types of invention, including chemical, mechanical, and electrical inventions. Microbiological inventions must therefore be fitted into this general framework as well as they can. Certain problems were bound to arise from the nature of living matter and it is also not surprising that attitudes towards what is patentable in this area can vary from one country to another.

Many of the ideas which have emerged in the experience of patenting chemical inventions, and the corresponding case law, have been extended to microbiological inventions. The most important of these is the distinction between process patents and product patents. Even for new chemical products many countries previously would only allow patents for particular processes of making these compounds and in many of the less-industrially developed countries this policy has not changed. Restricting the claims of a patent to a particular process has the consequence that third parties can devise alternative chemical routes to the same compounds which they will be legally free to use commercially. Allowing a claim for a new chemical compound *per se* means that no loophole is provided for someone who devises an alternative process and this gives the patentee much greater power in the market. This does not mean that an alternative process cannot be patented. If the alternative process is not obvious in view of the prior art existing at the date on which a patent application could be filed for the new process then it can usually be patented. This prior art might include the product patent and the process described in it, assuming this has been published, and any other published information which could be relevant in determining whether the alternative process involves an inventive step. However, the use of the alternative process is dominated by the earlier patent because the latter has the claim to the product *per se*. Therefore the use of the alternative process would require a licence under the product patent. This is an illustration of the principle stated in Chapter 1 that possession of a patent for any invention does not give its owner the automatic right to make or use the same but only to exclude others from doing so. Similarly, in the situation under discussion, if the owner of the earlier product patent wishes to switch to the alternative process he requires a licence from the owner of the later patent.

Even in some Western European countries unrestricted product claims for chemical compounds are still not available although those countries that join the European Patent Convention must eventually offer product patents of this type. These attitudes have been so strongly held in the past that they have carried over into the debate about the patentability of micro-organisms *per se* as distinct from particular processes for producing or for utilising micro-organisms. The economic consequences of allowing patents for micro-organisms are probably less important than those attaching to the granting of chemical product patents but the reluctance to allow product patents of this kind still exists in some countries.

In considering what is patentable in the area of biotechnology it is helpful to begin with classical biotechnology using fermentation methods and other processes to cultivate micro-organisms in order to produce microbial products which may be useful in themselves or, more usually, to produce useful by-products such as antibiotics, enzymes and vitamins. Then we must consider the newer biotechnology which has emerged over the last decade or more to produce new micro-organisms by direct genetic manipulation. Microbiological inventions of the classical type can be handled reasonably straightforwardly by applying the experience gained in handling chemical inventions. When defining a chemical process for the purposes of a patent claim it is necessary to specify the starting materials, the desired product, and the method or means by which the chemical conversion or treatment is achieved, e.g. by defining the reaction conditions or specifying the reagents or catalyst used. Two examples taken at random from the Official Gazette of the US Patent and Trademark Office are:

US Patent 4,331,592 (a chemical reaction process)
>   1. The method of making a carboxylic acid amide which comprises reacting a compound having a free amino group with a compound having a free carboxyl group in the presence of an anhydride of an alkane phosphonic acid.

US Patent 4,331,763 (a chemical extraction process)
>   1. A process for the production of ascorbate oxidase, comprising contacting plant tissue of the species *Sechium edule Sw.* with an aqueous alkaline medium as an extracting solvent, and separating ascorbate oxidase from the solvent solution thereof thus produced.

Microbiological processes can be described and defined in a similar way. Two more random examples are:

US Patent 4,634,670
>   1. A process for the preparation of cellulase in which a micro-organism of the genus *Trichoderma*, which is capable of producing cellulase, is cultured in order to accumulate cellulase in the culture medium and the resultant cellulase is harvested from the culture medium, characterised in that the said microorganism is a mutant strain of the genus *Trichoderma*, which exhibits increased inducibility of cellulase by L-sorbose relative to that of a given parent strain.

US Patent 4,626,430
>   1. A process for preparing a modified live *Pasteurella haemolytica* vaccine capable of inducing immunity in bovine, porcine and ovine animal species without serious side effects which comprises chemically modifying virulent *Pasteurella haemolytica* strain ATTC No. 31611 by passaging it in the presence of an acridinium salt and combining the modified bacteria with a carrier.

Where the micro-organism is a desired product of the process the patenting of the product is more difficult than in the corresponding

Table 6.1 *Patentable microbiological inventions*

(1) Process of producing a new micro-organism.
(2) The new micro-organism as produced by the defined process.
(3) The new micro-organism *per se*.
(4) Process of cultivating or otherwise using a known or a new micro-organism to produce an end-product which may be:
(a) a form of the multiplied micro-organism itself, for example vaccine or edible biomass;
(b) a by-product of microbial growth, for example an antibiotic, enzyme, toxin, or an otherwise useful industrial product (even if inactive biologically); or
(c) some other product or substrate which is produced or improved by the culturing process, for example a purified industrial product or effluent.
(5) The products of any of the processes defined in (4) – defined by a *per se* claim or product-by-process claim as appropriate.
(6) Particular formulations of defined strains or cultures thereof, including combinations with other substances, designed to utilise and exploit their special properties, for example, in human or animal foods or for industrial uses.

chemical case because of the problem of defining a product of such complex nature. This will be discussed below.

In the patenting of chemical inventions the kinds of patent that can be obtained are now fairly well established. For inventions in classical microbial biotechnology the main types of invention are shown in Table 6.1 in generalised form.

Inventions of the above kind have been the subject of considerable interest and discussion in patent circles and in the biotechnology research community for more than a decade. Three basic questions are:

(1)   Can you patent the micro-organism itself?

(2)   How do you define a micro-organism for purposes of a patent claim?

(3)   How can the inventor provide a patent disclosure which will enable others to repeat his work?

The first of these questions has attracted the widest scientific and public interest. In patent terms the question is whether a product *per se* claim to a micro-organism is allowable. The idea of patenting something living seems to have been more than a mere legal issue, perhaps a philosophical issue, on which international unanimity could not be expected immediately. Since patent laws are directed to articles of 'manufacture' or to 'compositions of matter' it was questionable at least in principle whether living organisms could come within these definitions. Against the view that you cannot patent 'life' it was pointed out that living organisms have increasingly become involved in modern industrial processes. Also, agriculture is as old as the hills. In the United States where the debate was fiercest the Supreme Court decided in 1980 in the Chakrabarty case to take the liberal view that anything under the sun is patentable if it meets the usual criteria and if human ingenuity and intervention have been necessary to produce it. 'Something pre-existing and merely plucked from the earth', as another lower US court put it, would not be patentable as a product *per se* but so long as human technical intervention is involved, by devising inventive methods of isolation or by modifying the form of the natural material in a useful way, there is no fundamental reason why patent protection should not be obtained. Even earlier, in Europe, the German Supreme Court had decided that there is nothing about biological inventions which removes them in principle from the sphere of patent protection so long as they have technical character and can be put into practice by the skilled worker from a technical description provided by the inventor.

It might be wondered why anyone would want to have protection for a micro-organism in the form of a *per se* claim of the kind mentioned above. On reason might be that the micro-organism has commercial importance in itself, e.g. as a vaccine strain or as a source of single cell protein where the micro-organism is contained in the commercial product. In some examples of this situation the patentee's product could be used by others as a starting point for their own manufacture and this would be a clear infringement of the micro-organism claim. More usually, the micro-organism is valuable primarily for what it produces, such as a secondary metabolite, and in this situation the following distinctions can be made. Where the micro-organism produces a novel product, e.g. an antibiotic it is usually straightfoward to obtain a *per se* product claim for what is going to be the marketed product and this gives the most commercially valuable type of protection. Along with such product claims it is customary also to have process claims covering the process for producing the product by means of the micro-organism. In these circumstances the main purpose of additional claims to the micro-organism *per se* will probably be as insurance against the possibility that the micro-organism will produce some other valuable product not yet discovered. Where the micro-organism produces a known product there will be no possibility of *per se* protection for that product but process claims for its production will be obtainable. Protection for the micro-organism *per se* will also be highly desirable as part of the same insurance policy mentioned above but also because such claims give the broadest protection that can be envisaged. Micro-organism claims may be quite useful when it comes to providing evidence or proof of infringement. In any event one should always seek maximum claim coverage both as to scope and type of patent claim in relation to an invention.

The second question, how to define a micro-organism, is one which inventors must themselves help to answer case by case. This question arises for process claims as well as product claims where the novel essential element is the micro-organism itself. Inventors would often like to define micro-organisms by their function or properties such as

> 'A strain of *Streptomyces aureofaciens* which produces tetracyclin to the substantial exclusion of chlortetracyclin'

but this would be regarded by Patent Offices usually as too imprecise or as merely stating a problem. Also, a broad functional statement of this kind could be said to be a mere statement of a concept which would be obvious to the skilled worker, in the sense that a strain having these properties would be an obviously desirable thing to possess.

Sometimes inventors may argue that the strains which have been discovered or developed are sufficiently different from the known species of a particular genus that they may themselves be regarded as a new species. From the scientific point of view such an assertion would have to be supported by appropriate microbiological criteria. But for patent law it is widely accepted that a specification can be its own 'dictionary' and that the inventor is therefore allowed to christen a group of strains by a new species name, e.g. *Micrococcus glutamicus*, so long as it is clear from the specification what are the distinguishing marks of this new species. The species name *Micrococcus glutamicus* was used in US Patent 3,003,925 being based on certain morphological and biochemical distinctions from previously known strains and also by the property of production in high yield of L-glutamate. This approach has received a setback however in United States patent practice by a decision of the Board of Appeals in a particular case in which the micro-organism was defined as

> 'A micro-organism belonging to the species *Micromonospora pilosospora* having the ability to produce antibiotic AX-127B-1'.

The applicant had developed three new strains having this common property and had deposited them in a culture collection and was therefore relying on a species name to cover also other strains not yet isolated or developed which would nevertheless have the same property. The Board held that the isolation and deposition of three strains would not enable the skilled worker to discover additional strains having the same property. Protection could only be allowed for the use of the three deposited strains.

Similarly, in the British Patent Office, an attempt to classify a single deposited strain as a new species *Micromonospora rosea species nova*, and to claim the micro-organism *per se*, was rejected. The British Patent

Office held that the applicant was not allowed to extrapolate from the single deposited strain and commented that in microbiological inventions it is not possible to allow predictive generalisation to the extent that this is possible for chemical inventions.

Where the invention is based on the utilisation of known micro-organisms there seems to be more latitude as regards the scope of definition. An early British patent in the biological detergent field, UK 1,243,784, contained the following claim:

> 'An enzyme preparation containing at least one proteolytic enzyme of the serine type produced by cultivation of species of the genus *Bacillus*, the said enzyme showing optimal proteolytic activity against hemoglobin in the presence of urea at a pH-value above 9.'

Claims of this type reciting the use of a whole genus are less easy to obtain nowadays but, to show the danger of making sweeping statements of this kind, a much more recently allowed US Patent No. 4,328,312 contains the following main process claim:

> 'A process for producing a peroxidase, which comprises culturing a micro-organism belonging to the genus *Myrothecium* and capable of producing a peroxidase in a nutrient medium, accumulating in the cultured product the peroxidase and collecting the accumulated peroxidase.'

It would be unwise to make comments about the scope of these claims without first reading the specification as a whole and perhaps also the history of the prosecution of the application in which the arguments for such broad definitions were advanced. A somewhat narrower approach is exemplified by US Patent 4,245,050 in which known species are recited as the source of a particular enzyme. The claim reads:

> 'A process for preparing choline oxidase which comprises culturing a microorganism belonging to the species *Brevibacterium album, Brevibacterium cerinum* or *Corynebacterium murisepticum* and being capable of producing choline oxidase when cultured in a nutrient medium accumulating choline oxidase in the culture liquor, and recovering said choline oxidase.'

The most usual form of definition, however, is one limited to the deposited strain, especially where claims to the micro-organism *per se* are presented, as in the following example of US Patent 4,329,432 which has the following product claim:

> 'A biologically pure culture of mutant *Mycobacterium fortuitum* NRRL B-8128.'

The enabling description of micro-organisms

In the discussion so far we have been concerned with the question of definition. Definition is necessary so that the scope of the patent is clear to the skilled worker from the legal standpoint. Now we must consider the more practical question of how the skilled person can reproduce the results described in the patent application. Where the invention depends upon a particular specified micro-organism, the micro-organism must be identified in the specification in order to disclose the invention in a manner sufficiently clear and complete for it to be carried out by a person skilled in the relevant art. Thus the inventor must provide an 'enabling disclosure'. If the micro-organism is a known strain available to the skilled worker it is sufficient to refer to it by name. But for a *new* micro-organism, the skilled person requires not only a description but also the means of access to the micro-organism. This problem became acute in the patenting of important post-war developments in antibiotics technology and it was solved by depositing new strains in culture collections from which they could be made available to those wishing to repeat the described processes. The maxim that what cannot be described must be deposited has since become fixed in patent law either by court decisions or by statute.

The deposition of micro-organisms for patent purposes

The practice of making so-called 'patent deposits' of micro-organisms first arose for inventions involving new strains isolated from soil or other sources or from mutation programmes. It is now so embedded in the thinking of many Patent Office officials that it continues to be raised in connection with new strains produced by genetic manipulation in spite of the fact that these techniques are more amenable to reproduction from a written description. The first legal decision on deposition was given in the United States of America in the celebrated Argoudelis case (these cases are usually referred to by name of inventor).

> *The Argoudelis application claimed two new antibiotics and a microbiological process for their production. The process involved a new* Streptomyces *strain which had been isolated from soil and deposited, before the filing of the US patent application, with a public depository in the USA. The micro-organism had been deposited under the condition that access to it would be restricted to persons authorised by the applicant in the period before the patent was granted. The US Patent Office had argued that this deposit was secret and confidential and therefore*

that the application was defective because the micro-organism had not been made available to the general public at the time of filing of the patent application. The Court held that it was not necessary for the public to have access to the culture before issuance of the patent. The applicant had set up a procedure whereby when the patent was granted others would have access to the deposited strain and so be able to reproduce the process. For many years after the Argoudelis decision it was assumed that the deposit would have to be made with the culture collection no later than the filing date of the patent application so that the latter could cross-refer to the deposited strain by its accession number. More recently this assumption has been modified by a US Court decision in the Lundak case where through oversight the patent application was made a little too soon, some days before the strain was deposited. The inventor, a university professor, argued that his cell line was effectively on deposit in the university laboratories and elsewhere and would therefore have been available to the Patent Office if required in examination of the application and accessible to the public from the culture collection on grant of the patent. The court agreed.

If deposition provides a legal solution of the description problem it does not necessarily provide a commercially acceptable solution. Deposition is required not merely to provide a reference material for Patent Office purposes but more importantly to enable samples to be made available to third parties. The main controversy on this issue is over the date of public release of the culture and the conditions that should be attached to this release. Under US patent law the situation, though not ideal, is generally acceptable whereas under the corresponding laws in European countries the timing and other conditions of release of samples of deposited micro-organisms are far from satisfactory to industry and other applicants for patents and are seen to disfavour the patent route as compared with the alternative of industrial secrecy. These views cannot be fully appreciated without referring again to the explanation of patent procedure and time-scale given in Chapter 5.

The scheme shown in Figure 4.8 (p. 59) indicates that a patent application is published in some countries while still at an early stage (18 months after the priority date). No official examination of its merits has yet begun. This is the norm in Europe under the EPC and most European national laws (also in Japan) but in USA publication does not occur until the patent is granted. The official view in Europe is that a published application is not an effective publication unless the deposited organism is made available at the same time.

Availability of deposited organisms

We have seen that, under US case law, general availability of the deposited strain is not required before the grant of a patent. In Europe, under the EPC, availability is covered by a specific regulation (Rule 28). Rule 28 requires an applicant to:

  (i)   deposit the new organism in an acceptable culture collection no later than the European patent application date

  (ii) quote the accession number of the deposited culture in the application

  (iii) accept that a sample of the deposited strain will be made available from the date of first publication to either (a) any person or (b) an independent expert nominated from an official list held by the European Patent Office. The function of the independent expert is to act for other persons or firms, e.g. the applicant's competitors, and to test, experiment with, and generally evaluate the invention on their behalf. The independent expert, though acting for third parties, must not pass the strain on to them. Under this alternative a measure of control on the use of the organism is provided for the applicant before he obtains an enforceable right.

Alternative (a) will apply unless the applicant opts for alternative (b) before preparations for publication of the application are complete. Availability under either (a) or (b) is subject to certain undertakings, namely

  (1)   While the patent application is pending or so long as the eventual patent lasts, the culture cannot be passed on to others by the person obtaining the sample from the culture collection.

  (2)   While the application is pending (but not after grant of the patent) the person obtaining the sample undertakes to use the culture for experimental purposes only.

Both undertakings cease upon refusal or withdrawal of the patent application.

Rule 28 also requires 'such relevant information as is available to the applicant on the characteristics of the micro-organism'. The European Patent Office guideline on this is reproduced as Appendix 5.

Rule 28 applies not only to the deposited micro-organism but also to cultures derived from the deposited organism and still exhibiting the characteristics of the deposited organism essential to carrying out the invention. This must include sub-cultures of the deposited strain and modifications thereof which meet the terms of the definition. It should be noted that the Rule applies only to micro-organisms not already available to the public 'and which cannot be described in the European patent application in such a manner as to enable the invention to be

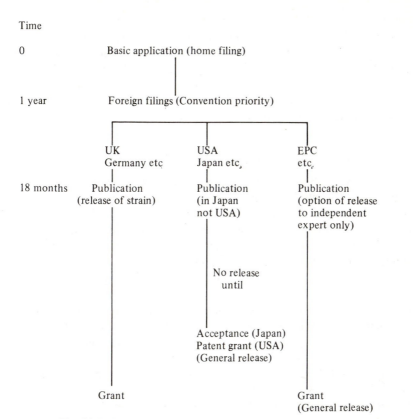

Fig. 6.1. Release of deposited strains.

carried out by a person skilled in the art'. This wording makes it possible to avoid depositing the new micro-organism where the applicant can describe a reproducible method of producing and identifying the micro-organism, e.g. by a repeatable technique of genetic manipulation.

The present situation on the release of deposited strains is summarised in Figure 6.1. UK and Germany are examples of countries which do not yet allow the independent expert option for national applications filed in their own countries, i.e. non-EPC applications, whereas the current EPC practice has been adopted by France and Scandinavian countries for national applications also.

Industry and other interested circles desire harmonisation of these varying practices in a way favourable to applicants by allowing for greater control over the precious new strain in the period before an enforceable right is obtained. The US and Japanese practices are the most favourable to applicants at the present time. European Patent Office practice is a compromise between, say, the US and UK systems but still far from ideal. Even after the grant of a patent there should be some restrictions on the availability of the deposited strain. For example, why should it be freely available in distant countries where no corresponding patent has been applied for? Should there not be a prohibition on exporting the strain to such a country? For some individual inventors and some industrial firms these drawbacks are a disincentive to patenting inventions of this kind.

International developments (The Budapest Treaty)

This is an international Convention governing the recognition of deposits in officially approved culture collections for the purposes of patent applications in any country that is a party to it. By the beginning of 1988 twenty two states had signed this Convention. According to the Budapest Treaty a culture collection may become designated as an International Depositary Authority (IDA) and thereby become recognised by all the contracting states. A single such depositary, whatever its location, can therefore be chosen by an applicant to hold a deposit relevant to a single patent application or to a family of related patent applications filed in any number of contracting states. An IDA must store a deposited micro-organism for at least 5 years after the most recent request for a sample and for at least 30 years from the original date of deposit. Eighteen IDAs now exist based in USA(3), UK(6), Bulgaria, France, West Germany, Hungary, Japan, Netherlands, and the Soviet Union (3) (See Glossary under Budapest Convention).

How to deposit

The full lists of contracting states and culture collections participating in the Budapest Treaty are given every year in the January issue of *'Industrial Property'* published by the World Intellectual Property Organisation based in Geneva. These lists identify the types of micro-organism accepted by each IDA and the fees for deposit. The depositor must provide information and data required by the IDA so that the deposit is effective for the purposes of the Treaty.

An inventor may require assistance from a culture collection and should certainly seek it especially to avoid errors of taxonomy. Corrections of errors of this kind have in the past been allowed in patent applications and patents when the scientific world itself recognised difficulties or disputes about naming micro-organisms. But a patentee cannot escape the consequences of the terms he uses to define an invention and Patent Offices will keep him to a tight rein on this in future. Where a micro-organism is defined in a patent by culture collection number it is arguable that the definition finally rests upon what has been deposited and not on how it has been named, but on such an important matter it is better to leave no argument open which could cause doubt.

How many strains must be deposited

This depends on the type of invention and especially on the scope of the patent claims. The narrower the invention the more reliance may be placed on the actual strains the inventor has worked on. The key issue in all questions about deposition is whether the written disclosure can be reproduced in an effective manner without access to the deposit. Therefore in the case of an invention which utilises a wide range of micro-organisms many of which are already known and available, one can say that a broad claim should be allowable without dependence on particular strains and in some cases no deposit will be necessary at all. However the specific detailed Examples included in the specification will (or should) describe actual experiments with particular strains and it may be necessary or desirable to deposit such strains in order to avoid all doubt about the reproducibility of this part of the disclosure. One also may wish to argue that the deposited strains are representative only, in which case it will be a matter of opinion how many are necessary to support the claim. This is a special example of the general principle that the disclosure must always be fairly commensurate with the scope of the protection being sought. These are primarily patent law problems upon which the inventor must be guided by the patent attorney, although it is as well for the experimental scientist to know the background. As a scientist he will also know that you cannot extrapolate from a single point!

The most usual problem under this heading is that the research worker will have studied a fairly small number of different strains and may have great difficulty in generalising from the data. This is a more fundamental question about the scope of the invention itself than one for consideration under the present heading alone. For the present, however, it can be said that where a number of strains have been found to be useful, whereas a number of related strains have not, the claim may have to list the successful strains and be limited by this list. In such a case the successful strains will require depositing. The only way out of this burden of effort and cost is to discover some common parameter of the useful strains which is related to performance and which enables further useful strains to be easily detected and discovered.

Products of Nature

Can you patent something that already exists in Nature, whether it be an inanimate chemical compound, an enzyme, a micro-organism or higher life form, or a gene? These items are given in this sequence because this is the chronological order in which the parts of this question have arisen either for the courts or for the patent lawyer advising his client. In the past patents certainly have been granted for isolated vitamins, hormones, steroids, alkaloids and other substances but biotechnology has given new life to this controversial subject.

The question raises more than one issue. Patents are concerned with the economic life of man and the bringing into being of what is useful in an economic context. As regards its utility to man there is no reason why research into natural products should be treated differently from research in other areas of chemistry. Therefore there ought to be no preconceived idea in legal thinking which would exclude patent protection for natural substances simply because they exist in the first place. Yet at various levels of the patent system, from the judiciary downwards, the notion that the works of Nature must be left open to all free from any constraints is very persistent. For example, many years ago the US Supreme Court, in rejecting a patent for certain bacterial inoculants used for nitrogen fixation, referred to the particular invention patented as 'no more than the discovery of some of the handiwork of nature and hence not patentable'. It is in the United States that this attitude is most prevalent. In Europe there is more flexibility and a greater willingness to re-examine the issues in the light of modern biotechnology.

The product of Nature problem is also compounded by the fact that most patent laws make a distinction between 'discovery' and 'invention' and exclude *mere* discovery from the benefit of patent protection. This distinction is seized upon by those who would argue that the isolation of substances from Nature is mere discovery and therefore unpatentable. This argument is buttressed by appeal to the novelty requirement in patent law; it is said that the natural product previously existed, therefore it is old, therefore it cannot be new, therefore it cannot be patented, q.e.d.

No patent statute uses the term 'old' as opposed to 'new'. The test for novelty in US patent law is applied in relation to what was 'known or used by others' before the applicant made the invention for which he is seeking patent protection. The test also applies to what has been 'patented or described in a printed publication' before the applicant's invention date or more than one year before his application date in the United States. Under the European patent convention the test for novelty is applied to the so-called 'state of the art' which comprises 'everything made available to the public . . . before the date of filing of the European patent application'. In both United States and European patent law, therefore, it is apparently the assumption that the relevant knowledge or thing must be already in the possession of the public in order to constitute prior art. This knowledge can be by way of publication in the ordinary accepted sense or by prior use.

The European test for novelty is founded on the concept of prior availability to the public. There is perhaps an element of ambiguity in the term 'available'. Most things are available for discovery if only we have the brains or the luck to actually make the discovery. Products of Nature are therefore 'available' in this broad sense but the law cannot be given such an absurd interpretation. The moon has always been available to mankind but a great deal of effort and ingenuity was necessary before man could handle moondust. Likewise natural products are usually inaccessible in nature and have to be spotted, dug-out, and identified. Perhaps the European Patent Office Guidelines have this in mind when they refer to *free* occurrence in the following extract:

> 'To find a substance freely occurring in Nature is also mere discovery and therefore unpatentable. However, if a substance found in nature has first to be isolated from its surroundings and a process for obtaining it is developed, that process is patentable. Moreover, if the substance can be properly characterised either by its structure, by the process by which it is obtained or by other parameters and it is "new" in the absolute sense of having no previously recognised existence, then the substance per se may be patentable. An example of such a case is that of a new substance which is discovered as being produced by a micro-organism.'

In 1980 the United States Supreme Court allowed US Patent 4,259,444 to A. Chakrabarty with the following claim:

> 'A bacterium from the genus *Pseudomonas* containing therein at least two stable energy-generating plasmids, each of said plasmids providing a separate hydrocarbon degradative pathway.'

This bacterium was a manipulated oil-degrading organism. The court said that 'a new mineral discovered in the earth or a new plant found in the wild is not patentable subject matter'. But here the claim was not to a hitherto unknown natural phenomenon but to 'a non-naturally occurring manufacture or composition of matter, a product of human ingenuity having a distinctive known character and use'. In also rejecting the product of Nature argument the court held that the patentee had produced a new bacterium with markedly different characteristics from any found in Nature and one having the potential for significant utility. This was not Nature's handiwork but that of the inventor.

The important distinction made in the Chakrabarty case continues to be applied by the US Patent Office. Therefore as far as naturally occurring organisms are concerned these cannot be claimed without some further restriction. In practice US patents for these are now regularly limited to 'biologically pure cultures' of the specified organism. This practice was approved by a lower US court which stated that while 'something pre-existing and merely plucked from the earth and claimed as such' could not be patented this was 'a far cry from a biologically pure culture produced by great labor in a laboratory and so claimed'.

Mutants and variants

It is usually possible to overcome a product of Nature objection to a claim for a micro-organism, or even a higher organism, if what is claimed is a mutant form which has arisen in the laboratory either by chance or by design. It is assumed that under laboratory conditions continued subculture or more drastic treatment of a naturally occurring organism has given rise to something 'new' as a result of human technical intervention. Where the method for producing specific mutants can be described it will be possible to obtain product claims to these as, for example, the following:

US 4,324,860

> A biologically pure culture of a mutant of *Streptococcus mutans* strain BHT-2 (str) having a single point mutation in the structural gene for lactate dehydrogenase, being gram positive, having spheroidal cells occurring in pairs and chains and producing on glucose tetrazolium medium bright red colonies of relatively larger size than those produced by the parent strain.

But in any patent for a naturally occurring micro-organism produced by isolation or for a mutant form of such it may be desirable for the claim to cover further 'mutants or variants thereof'. It is not always possible to obtain claims of this rather open-ended sort, especially if no examples of such related organisms can be given in the specification. The practice varies from country to country and it would be dangerous to attempt a summary of what is likely to vary further as patent practice develops.

The courts could overcome this problem to a marked extent by holding that so long as there is derivation from the patented organism and so long as the original properties are retained in the derived organism then the latter is still covered by the patent. Even if the derived organism shows some additional property or improvement which makes it patentable over the parent organism the idea of a 'dependent patent' has existed in patent law for a long time and would apply comfortably to this situation. Rule 28 discussed earlier in this chapter (p. 84) is already familiar with the question of derived cultures although the Rule 28 context is procedural rather than one of substantive law.

Proteins, enzymes, antigens, antibodies

This is a convenient point at which to consider how proteins and other biologically active substances of high molecular weight are handled patentwise. Substances in this group may be produced by microbiological cultivation or often by extraction from plant and animal cells and tissues in which they are found in Nature. The basic question here is how these are to be covered by product claims preferably of the *per se* type whenever possible. In other words how are these products to be defined?

The approach of the patent attorney to the characterisation of products of this type for patent purposes is inevitably coloured by experience in the patenting of simpler chemical compounds. In chemistry the attorney is accustomed to more structural precision at the molecular level and from this habit of thought attorneys, and Patent Office Examiners also, will look for chemical definition based on the structural formula of the compound. With larger molecules such as synthetic polymers it is recognised that the products are rarely homogeneous as to molecular size and are usually mixtures of species of varying chain length. The common feature of this mixture is the repeating structural unit derived from the monomer or monomers used and the resulting polymer can therefore be specified in terms of the repeating unit and a range of molecular weight. For a polypeptide the complete amino acid sequence would provide a definition which would most satisfy the general organic chemist. The protein chemist and the biologist will be much more accustomed to thinking about biological function and will regard the amino acid sequence as an oversimplification when it comes to providing a definition. The enzyme cholesterol oxidase can be obtained from species of micro-organism from different genera including *Nocardia, Streptomyces* and *Brevibacterium*. The chemist will ask 'But is it the same enzyme?' and the biochemist will answer affirmatively yet in the full knowledge that there will be differences of molecular weight and amino acid composition as between cholesterol oxidase from these different sources. One might well ask what objection there could be to defining a new product solely in terms of biological function. At one time the answer would be that for the purposes of a patent claim one must define a substance in terms of what it is rather than what it does. But as more biological products of this general kind are becoming the subject of patents there is now a trend towards placing much greater reliance on the statement of biological properties. Could this be done for an enzyme? We have seen earlier in this chapter examples of enzyme patents where the claim defines the enzyme by reference to the microbial source from which it is produced. This is the normal sort of definition where the enzyme is not fundamentally new but has improved activity or other properties which derive from its particular source. The Japanese Patent Office guidelines are quite specific in requiring or strongly recommending that an enzyme be claimed by reference to the following 11 items of which the first three are considered the most important:

 (1)   Activity
 (2)   Specificity on substrate
 (3)   Optimum pH range and stable pH range
 (4)   Determination method for potency
 (5)   Range of temperature appropriate for activity
 (6)   Condition of deactivation due to pH, temperature, etc.
 (7)   Inhibition, activation and stabilisation
 (8)   Purification method
 (9)   Molecular weight
(10)   Crystal structure
(11)   Elementary analysis

Where the enzyme is fundamentally new in the sense that the particular enzymatic reaction is not to be found in the prior literature some quite broad definitions are possible as shown in the following two U.S. patents.

US 4,202,941

> Glycerol oxidase characterised by its ability to oxidize glycerol in the presence of oxygen to form hydrogen peroxide and glyceraldehyde.

US 4,255,519

> 1. An oxidizing enzyme of glycerol having the following properties:
>   (1)   action: oxidizes glycerol in the presence of oxygen to form hydrogen peroxide and glyceraldehyde;
>   (2)   substrate specificity: a specific activity for glycerol and dihydroxyacetone;
>   (3)   optimum pH: 7.8–8.6;
>   (4)   stable pH: 7.5–10.0;
>   (5)   optimum temperature for action: 37°C; and
>   (6)   Michaelis constant against glycerol (K_m value): 8.0×10^{-3} M.

The first of these two patents covers the whole family of enzymes having the stated properties. The oxidase was first isolated from various species of *Aspergillus* and *Neurospora*. The second patent describes the isolation of the enzyme from a *Penicillium* species and claims the specific enzyme in terms of the data given. The second patent refers to this enzyme as glycerol oxidase II and describes the enzyme of the first patent as glycerol oxidase I.

Two more examples of enzyme patents are the following.

US 4,536,477

> A glucoamylase enzyme derived from a *Clostridium thermoamylolyticum* microorganism, said enzyme having a molecular weight of about 75.000 ± 3.000 as determined by SDS–polyacrylamide gel electrophoresis, having a half-life of greater than 3 hours at pH 6 and 70 °C, having a maximum glucoamylase activity at a pH of about 5.0, and having a maximum glucoamylase activity at pH 5 at a temperature of about 70–75 °C.

US 4,386,160

> A thermally destabilized *Bacillus* serine protease acylated with an acylating derivative of a monocarboxylic acid containing about 1 to 6 carbon atoms to a reduced thermal stability of at least about 3 °C at pH 7.5 and having at least about 50% of the proteolytic activity before acylating.

Where enzymes are extracted from venoms and animal tissues a common form of claim which can be used is one which specifies the venom or tissue source, states the activity of the enzyme, and follows with a combination of physicochemical characteristics including electrophoretic mobility, isoelectric point, sedimentation coefficient, molecular weight, extinction coefficient and other items. One example of this is given in detail in the case study in Chapter 10. Further examples of claims to substances of this general kind are given below.

US 4,500,451

> A new placental protein PP_{13} extracted from human placental tissue characterized by the following:
> (a) an electrophoretic mobility in the same range as albumin,
> (b) an isoelectric point of 4.75 ± 0.15,
> (c) a sedimentation coefficient $S_{20}0_w$ of 3.1 ± 0.15,
> (d) a molecular weight determined by ultracentrifugation of 30,000 ± 5,000,

(e)   a molecular weight determined in polyacrylamide gel containing sodium dodecyl sulphate (SDS) of 29,000 ± 3,000,

(f)   an extinction coefficient $E_{1cm}1\%$ (280 nm) of 9.8 ± 0.3 and

(g)   a carbohydrate content of 1% (0.1 ± 0.05% mannose, 0.2 ± 0.1% galactose, 0.1 ± 0.05% xylose, 0.2 ± 0.1% glucosamine, and neuraminic acid not detected).

US 4,376,071

A substantially purified proteinaceous factor obtained from spinal cord which has mitogenic activity, a molecular weight of about 11,000, a pI of 9.6 and which is heat and acid labile.

US 4,383,985

Breast cancer antigens, designated "BCA", and characterized as follows:

(a)   being endogenous to and extractable with a glycoprotein solvent from human primary breast carcinomas,

(b)   unreactive with carcinoembryonic antigen antiserum,

(c)   reactive only with antiserum produced by antigens extracted from human primary breast carcinomas, and

(d)   essentially free of other endogenous material.

US 4,544,640

An anti-immune complex antibody, which is a glycoprotein having a molecular weight of from 150,000 to 180,000 as determined by gel filtration, reacts with an immune complex in a blood serum of a human patient having systemic lupus erythematosus, rheumatoid arthritis or tetanus, and which does not react with aggregated IgG.

US 4,559,230

A glycoprotein having a molecular weight of about 14,000 daltons and an isoelectric point of about 4.6; a 1 mg/ml aqueous solution of said glycoprotein having an absorportion of ϵ = 0.12 units of optical density at 280 nm; said glycoprotein being isolated by a process comprising:

(a)   admixing pollen of *Dactylis glomerata* with an aqueous medium, thereby extracting water-soluble products;

(b)   separating the aqueous extract from insoluble matter;

(c)   subjecting said aqueous extract to fractionation by
molecular weight and isoelectric point; and

(d)   isolating said glycoprotein.

US 4,544,500

An antigen comprising a foot-and-mouth disease virus mono-
specific synthetic antigenic determinant peptide having about
twenty amino acids corresponding to a twenty amino acid
sequence of the foot-and-mouth disease virus protein VP_1 in the
130 to 160 region.

Viruses and vaccines

The patenting of a virus raises no legal issue beyond those already
discussed for micro-organisms and products of Nature. The first question
will therefore be whether the virus is new in the sense of having been
isolated for the first time, or new because it is a modified form of the
wild type. How the virus can be characterised for the purpose of a claim
is best dealt with case by case, and there are not so many precedents as
for bacteria by way of guidance. The utility of the virus will also have to
be considered. The most usual utility is as a vaccine strain and there is
no difficulty in principle about obtaining a claim to a vaccine containing
virus X (or any other antigen) as an antigenic component. A vaccine
claim usually implies the presence of a diluent or carrier and this is
sometimes stated in the claim, but this is not always essential. One
example of a patent for a virus and a virus vaccine is given as case study
2 in Chapter 10.

> *A recent important case decided by the Federal German
> Supreme Court involved a claim to a novel form of rabies virus
> as follows:*
> *'Rabies virus (nov. spec.) Strain 675, deposited at the
> Czechoslovakian national culture collection, Institute for
> Hygiene and Epidemiology, Prague, Registration No. CNCTC
> AO 4/77, obtainable by multiplication of HEP-flury-vaccine in
> primary or secondary spf-chicken embryo fibroplasts or in other
> rabies virus receptive cell lines or diploid cell genus, isolation of
> a plaque which differs in comparison with the starting virus by its
> intensified cytopathic effect in the plaque test, and cloning this
> plaque through three plaque passages, and characterized by the
> following features:*
> *(a)   very pronounced cell destroying cytopathic effect (cpE)
> in cell cultures, which differs distinctly from the cpE
> caused by the starting virus;*

(b) *a reduced primary virus cycle of 9 to 11 hours in
     comparison to the starting virus;*

(c) *very clear plaques, the average diameter of which is
     1 mm larger than the diameter of the plaques of the
     starting virus;*

(d) *faster induction of the interferon production in vivo
     after vaccination;*

(e) *increased infection titer in cell cultures in comparison
     with the starting virus;*

*as well as its mutants or variants with the same reproducible
significant cpE as well as the other specific charcteristics of Strain
675.*

   *The Supreme Court reversed its previous rulings, under the
older German law, that reproducibility of the patent description,
for a product claim, could not be achieved by use of the deposit
system and had to be self-contained in the application alone. The
Court took the opportunity under the 1978/1981 Patent Acts to
bring German jurisprudence into line with the practice of the
European Patent Office in this respect so that throughout Europe
there is now unanimity on the effectiveness of a culture collection
deposit of a micro-organism in supplementing the written patent
description for both process patents and product patents.*

The 'product of Nature' question continues to be a point of difficulty in
patent law. In the older case law, the question arose in connection with
the isolation of relatively simple naturally occurring compounds, e.g.
adrenalin, Vitamin B_{12} and certain steroids. In its modern context, it
re-surfaces in relation to the patentability of natural proteins purified
and isolated for the first time in quantity from cell culture systems or
from genetically programmed organisms. It is also involved in the
intriguing question of the patentability of natural gene sequences.
Questions of this type are now common in the field of the new
biotechnology, which is the subject of the next chapter.

7　The new biotechnology

The previous chapter dealt with what might be termed classical biotechnology. For the patenting of inventions in the new biotechnology, which includes recombinant DNA methods and cell fusion methods to produce hybridomas and other organisms, most of what has been said in the previous chapter is relevant here also. But the complexities of these new techniques for gene splicing or cell fusion, and the particular biological entities they make use of, give rise to additional categories of patentable invention. A comprehensive review of the possibilities would require a major work beyond the scope of this chapter and no attempt will be made here to give more than an outline and brief selection of patents actually granted so far. Most of the examples given are taken from United States patents which have issued in relatively large numbers since the first recombinant DNA patent was granted in December 1980. Some are chosen because of their commercial significance, some at random.

Genetic engineering methods and strategies

The Cohen-Boyer Patent

The first United States recombinant DNA patent granted was US 4,237,224 issued to inventors S.N. Cohen and H.W. Boyer and their assignee (the registered owner of the patent) the Board of the University of Stanford. The University administers the patent and has granted a large number of licences which return significant royalty income for the support of University work. The first claim of this patent is rather lengthy in wording but it boils down to a method involving the following series of steps:-

    (a)   Cleaving viral or plasmid DNA to form a first segment with an intact replicon

    (b)   Combining the first segment with a second DNA segment containing a gene which is foreign to a given unicellular organism

(the first or second segment containing a gene for a phenotypical trait)

    (c)   Transforming the unicellular organism with the functional DNA produced in (b)

(d)   Isolating transformant organisms by means of the phenotypical trait.

This claim and the 10 following claims cover a basic technique used in the laboratory to prepare recombinant organisms which can be cultivated so as to express the foreign gene and produce foreign protein. The actual step of producing the foreign protein product is specified in Claims 12 to 14.

The second Cohen-Boyer patent US 4,339,538, also deriving from the original application that resulted in the first patent, is directed to various recombinant molecules for which the following claim is general:

> 1. As a composition of matter, a biologically functional recombinant plasmid capable of selection and replication in a unicellular microorganism cell comprising: a first DNA segment containing an intact replicon recognized by said cell derived by cleaving a virus or plasmid compatible with said cell at other than the replicon site, which segment is covalently joined *in vitro* at its ends to the complementary ends of a second DNA segment foreign to said cell having at least one intact gene, said second DNA segment derived from a source which does not exchange genetic information with said cell.

As the contents of these two patents are concerned with the basic methodology used in the laboratory it was necessary in devising a licensing strategy to cater for the variety of applications of these techniques and the various types of intermediate and final product which can result from their use.

The Axel et al. Patent

US Patent 4,339,216 held on behalf of Columbia University shows a variation on the basic Cohen-Boyer technique in which the selectable phenotype DNA does not have to be linked directly to either of the two fragments which are spliced together in the basic method. This technique is limited to the genetic manipulation of eucaryotic cells, which apparently have the property of taking up all the available DNA under certain conditions. This is expressed in the claim as follows:

> 'A process for inserting foreign DNA I into a suitable eucaryotic cell which comprises cotransforming said eucaryotic cell with said foreign DNA I and with unlinked foreign DNA II which codes for a selectable phenotype not expressed by said eucaryotic cell, said cotransformation being carried out under suitable conditions permitting survival or identification of eucaryotic cells which have acquired said selectable phenotype, said foreign DNA I being incorporated into the chromosomal DNA of said eucaryotic cell.'

Vectors

The most common vectors to be patented, or described in genetic
engineering patents, are plasmids. Plasmids, being DNA molecules, are
patentable as chemical compounds but as such they require to be
characterised. The form of claim for a plasmid will depend on whether it
is a naturally occurring or a recombinant plasmid. The first recombinant
plasmid patent obtained in the United States is US 4,339,538 mentioned
in the previous section. The claim which has been set out above is one of
the most general of its kind. Since then the most usual form of patent
claim for a plasmid relies on a code name together with a restriction
map.

US Patent 4,273,875 covers a plasmid isolated from a naturally
occurring micro-organism. The micro-organism is described as novel but
nevertheless the claim to it, set out below, is limited to the pure culture.
This limitation was also considered necessary for the claim to the
plasmid. The two sample claims are:

> 1. Essentially pure plasmid pUC6 which is characterized by a
> molecular weight of approximately 6.0 megadaltons, and a
> restriction endonuclease cleavage map as shown in the drawing.
> 2. A biologically pure culture of *Streptomyces espinosus* biotype
> 23724A, having the deposit accession number NRRL 11439,
> and which also contains about 20 to about 40 copies of plasmid
> pUC6 per cell.

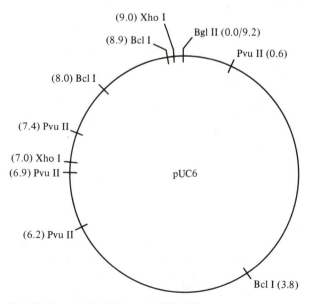

Fig. 7.1. Drawing for US Patent 4, 273, 875.

Some US patents have been granted with broad claims to recombinant plasmids and other vectors defined in terms of the added DNA, i.e. the gene insert, or its expression product. A good example of variations on this theme is US Patent 4,332,499 which has the following claims:

1. A recombinant DNA plasmid or bacteriophage transfer vector comprising a cDNA sequence comprising the endorphin gene cDNA sequence.

2. The transfer vector of claim 1 wherein the cDNA sequence comprises cDNA coding for the amino acid sequence:
Pro-Tyr-Arg-Val-Glu-His-Phe-Arg-Trp-Ser-Asn-Pro-Pro-Lys-Asp-Lys-Arg-Tyr-Gly-Gly-Phe-Met-Thr-Ser-Glu-Lys-Ser-Gln-Thr-Pro-Leu-Val-Thr-Leu-Phe-Lys-Asn-Ala-Ile-Ile-Lys-Asn-Ala-His-Lys-Lys-Gly.

3. The transfer vector of claim 1 comprising the cDNA sequence: 5'-
GG CCC TAC CGG GTG GAG CAC TTC CGC TGG AGC
AAC CCG CCC AAG GAC AAG CGT TAC GGT TTC
ATG ACC TCC GAG AAG AGC GAG ACG CCC CTG
GTG ACG CTC TTC AAG AAC GCC ATC ATC AAG
AAC CGC CAC AAG AAG GGC C-3'.

4. A microorganism transformed by the transfer vector of claim 1.

5. A microorganism transformed by the transfer vector of claim 2.

6. The plasmid pBR-322/ME-150.

7. Bacteria transformed by the plasmid of claim 6.

8. The microorganism *E. coli* χ1776-ME-150.

This is another patent to emanate from a University team, the University of California at Berkeley, and is based on the isolation of messenger RNA and the synthesis of the corresponding cDNA using reverse transcriptase followed by cloning of this sequence. This patent does not contain a claim to the cDNA sequence *per se* and there may be good reasons for its absence. In general, however, it is worth noting that cDNA does not exist in nature and we can expect to find claims of this type in appropriate circumstances.

Three more interesting claims to vectors are given below, the third being of interest in plant genetic manipulation:

US 4,510,245

A yeast expression vector comprising a replication origin functional in yeast and a DNA coding segment and an adenovirus major late promoter segment adjacent to the 5' end of the coding segment, the promoter segment being oriented so as to initiate transcription of the coding segment.

US 4,546,082

A DNA expression vector capable of expressing in yeast cells a product which is secreted from said yeast cells, said vector comprising at least a segment of alpha-factor precursor gene and at least one segment encoding a polypeptide.

US 4,536,475

A vector precursor comprising the Pst I cleaved left and right border fragments of the T region of the TI plasmid *Agrobacterium tumefaciens* strain of C58 interligated and ligated into the Pst I site of plasmid pBR322.

Two examples of phage vectors with representative claims are:

US 4,332,897

1. A temperate-bacteriophage whose DNA molecule is endonuclease-sensitive only in the DNA region carrying genetic information for the production of coat proteins.
9. A method for preparing a novel bacteriophage, which comprises making a bacteriophage of the lambdoid phage species endonuclease-resistant and mating the resulting bacteriophage with a lambdoid phage having endonuclease-sensitivity in the DNA region carrying genetic information for the production of coat proteins to obtain a bacteriophage having endonuclease-sensitivity only in the DNA region carrying genetic information for the production of coat proteins.

US 4,332,901

A cloning vector for use in recombining DNA which is a mutant of bacteriophage P4 wt or P4 vir$_1$ characterized in that it has plaque forming units appearing, in a cesium chloride equilibrium density gradient at 24 °C., in the density range from 1.42 to 1.35 g/ml and displaying a density profile of plaque forming units having three peaks at about 1.42, 1.39 and 1.35 g/ml respectively.

An important patent which covers the use of cosmids, as defined in its main method claim, is:

US 4,304,863

Process for the production of hybrid bacteria, characterized in that

(a)   a hybrid plasmid having only one cos site of a lambda or a lambdoid phage is produced from (1) a bacterial plasmid of not more than 21 Megadaltons and having only one cos site of a lambda or a lambdoid phage and (2) a foreign DNA fragment,

(b)   the resulting hybrid plasmid is packaged with the lysate of a lambda or lambdoid phage and

(c)   the packaging product is transduced into *Escherichia coli* whereby hybrid bacteria are formed.

It is important to note that this patent does not cover cosmids as such. Therefore the sale of cosmids would not be a direct infringement of the patent. However US law on infringement also embraces indirect infringement where a product is sold with the intention or knowledge that it will be used for the process claimed in the patent. This is known as 'contributory infringement'. The unlicensed sale of cosmids could therefore in certain circumstances be a contributory infringement and in any event the purchaser of a cosmid would not be free to use it to construct hybrid bacteria without a licence (direct or indirect) from the patentee. Infringement is discussed further in Chapter 9.

Patenting genes and gene products

The DNA sequence constituting a particular gene is an inanimate chemical substance which at first sight ought to be patentable as a chemical compound. In so far as the particular gene, in the form in which it has to be claimed, is a naturally occurring substance this question raises again the 'product of nature' complication. To the extent that any biological property is attributable to a particular gene or combination of genes it is known in principle that the gene(s) for such a property must exist. To seek and find and identify such genes might therefore appear as an obviously desirable thing to do first for scientific purposes and secondly for possible commercial reasons. However to achieve these objectives and to take the next step of cloning the gene in such a way that it will be successfully expressed cannot be dismissed so lightly. This work will frequently involve great experimental difficulty and its success may depend on a combination of skill and luck which is a hallmark of an inventive advance in the art. The question of patentability is therefore by no means easy for the patent lawyer. The question is now being faced by Patent Office Appeal Boards and Courts of Law in various countries in connection with disputes between commercial firms. These inevitably take time to resolve as neither side will give up without a struggle or forego any chance of appeal against an adverse decision.

Before a case comes into court the patent must have been granted by the Patent Office. Most Patent Offices have foreseen these legal difficulties and some have established their own viewpoint as to what is patentable in the general area of genetic engineering. The Japanese Patent Office has been the first in suggesting informal guidelines for applicants in this field as they have done more formally for applicants in other areas of technology (see extract in Appendix 5). The European Patent Office has not issued a formal guideline but has made its policy widely known. So far the most important common feature of European and Japanese practice is the reluctance to allow a claim of the broad functional type, for example,

'A nucleotide sequence coding for polypeptide X'.

Where X is a known peptide such claims would usually be rejected. Where X is new they may be allowed. These claims become more acceptable however if either the base sequence of the DNA or the amino acid sequence of the peptide is specified. The reader should note the cautious way in which these statements have to be made at present in a period of development of the official practice for inventions of this kind.

The US Patent Office have not issued any statements in the nature of a guideline but, as will be clear from the numerous examples quoted from US patents, one can make deductions as to what may succeed. The following example is instructive; the fragment defined does not exist as such in nature.

US 4,511,652

A DNA sequence encoding yeast copper chelatin or a copper chelating fragment thereof having naturally occurring flanking regions, each flanking region being less than 5 kbp.

One may ask whether the patenting of genes is more a matter of academic professional interest than one of real commercial importance. The genes as such would be rather unusual articles of commerce. For practical purposes it is usually the expression product or some derivative of this which is to be made and sold on a commercial scale. One major exception to this rule is a genetically manipulated plant where the gene is retained in the final product. But this special topic is reserved for the next chapter. This greater emphasis on the final product is shown in the UK patent for human tissue plasminogen activator which is the subject of current litigation. A brief account of the present state of the case is given below.

UK Patent 2,119,804

This patent issued with a series of broad product claims to human TPA in forms other than the naturally occurring substance. The following selection of claims shows the various ways in which the product was covered. It shows also the claims to vectors and transformed micro-organisms. The nature of the process used to make this product is very broadly defined in Claim 17.

1. Recombinant human tissue plasminogen activator essentially free of other proteins of human origin.

2. Human tissue plasminogen activator unaccompanied by associated native glycosylation.

3. Human tissue plasminogen activator as produced by recombinant DNA technology.

4. Biologically active human tissue plasminogen activator in essentially pure form, unaccompanied by protein with which it is ordinarily associated.

5. Human tissue plasminogen activator per se, of the kind produced by expression of a recombinant DNA sequence coding therefor in a mammalian cell line.

6. Human tissue plasminogen activator according to claims 1–5 containing a sequence of a polypeptide preceding the N-terminus of the first amino acid of said human tissue plasminogen activator.

7. A recombinant cloning vector comprising a DNA sequence encoding human tissue plasminogen activator.

8. A replicable expression vector capable, in a transformant microorganism or cell culture, of expressing a DNA sequence according to claim 7.

9. The plasmid p△RIPA° or pt-PAtrp12.

10. A microorganism or cell culture transformed with the vehicle according to claim 8 or 9.

17. A process for producing human t-PA, which process comprises:

   (a)   preparing a replicable expression vector capable of expressing the DNA sequence encoding human t-PA in a host cell;

   (b)   transforming a host cell culture to obtain a recombinant host cell;

   (c)   culturing said recombinant host cells under conditions permitting expression of said t-PA encoding DNA sequence to produce human t-PA;

   (d)   recovering said human t-PA.

In the court of first instance it was held that these broad product claims would only have been acceptable if the patentee had been the first to discover TPA or its desirable properties. Although the patentee had been the first to identify the DNA coding sequence and to deduce the amino acid sequence of the protein it had already been accepted by other workers as desirable to produce TPA in quantity by recombinant DNA methods. These product claims were therefore too wide in being directed to an obviously desirable and potentially possible end reached by routes on which only limited guidance had been given. This decision is under appeal. It must be emphasised that it is premature to draw any general significance from it. The case was one relating to a naturally occurring protein which was known to exist and had previously been isolated from cells in which it is normally produced in nature. It was specifically said that if the patentee had produced a new and valuable variant of TPA then protection for that might have been possible. It follows that protein engineering, i.e. adapting recombinant methods to produce new proteins, should receive more sympathetic treatment under patent law.

Hybridoma technology

The patenting of hybridomas and other cell lines is based on the principles established for micro-organism patents.

Spleen cells (lymphocytes) taken from an experimental animal immunised with a particular antigen are fused with cells of a tumour cell line (myeloma) derived from an animal of the same or a related type and from the resulting hybrid cells (hybridomas) there is selected the particular hybridoma clone which retains the property of selective antibody formation against a single particular antigen (monoclonal antibody). This hybridoma is itself a new cell line or clone. Inventions of this kind offer the possibility of claims to any novel parent myeloma utilised, claims to a family of derived hybridomas and to specific hybridomas, and claims to the production of monoclonal antibodies in process or product terms, as well as claims to applications of these in therapy or diagnostics.

After the publication in 1975 of the basic Milstein/Köhler technique and the subsequent appreciation of its more general importance it was reasonable to assume that the patentability of any application of this general procedure must rest on some special and non-obvious property or advantage of the particular system constructed, in much the same way as should apply to the patenting of particular applications of recombinant DNA methodology. Mere novelty should not be enough.

In view of the great variety of antigens, new hybridomas are now being produced in their thousands and many of them do not justify the cost of patenting. Myeloma parent strains with particular advantages are clearly worth patenting because they are intermediates for the production of an unlimited number of distinct hybridomas. For these myelomas the requirement of deposition with consequential availability of the cell line is acceptable in many cases. Many hybridomas tend to be retained as secret know-how as they cannot be 'reverse engineered' from their antibodies, the latter being most usually the marketed product.

The examples given below begin with the development of the first rat myeloma cell line suitable as a fusion partner while the second relates to an even further improvement on the original in that it lacks the ability to express any immunoglobulin chain. The designation numbers given are those by which the cell lines are referred to in the official culture collection held by the Pasteur Institute.

US 4,350,683

1. A substantially pure rat myeloma cell line having the C.N.C.M. designation I-078.
2. A hybrid cell line prepared from cells of the cell line C.N.C.M. I-078 through the fusion thereof with immunocyte cells from an animal sensitized to an immunogen in a nutrient medium for said cells, followed by isolation of the hybrid cell line from the resultant mixture of cells.

US 4,472,500

1. The rat myeloma cell line YB2/3.0 Ag.20.
2. A rat myeloma cell line being a variant of the cell line YB2/3.0.Ag.20 prepared by passaging and/or cloning cell line YB2/3.0.Ag.20.
3. A hybrid myeloma cell line derived from a parent myeloma cell line according to claim 1 or 2.

The next two examples do not refer in the claim to a deposit number.

US 4,514,498

A composition of matter consisting essentially of a continuous murine hybrid cell line that produces monoclonal antibody against an antigenic determinant of *Treponema pallidum*, which cell line is formed as a fusion between a murine myeloma cell and a differentiated murine lymphoid cell immunized with *Treponema pallidum* antigen.

US 4,491,632

A composition comprising a hybrid continuous cell line that produces antibody to a viral hepatitis antigen which comprises a cell hybrid of an animal spleen cell immunized with viral hepatitis antigen fused to a myeloma derived from the same animal species as the spleen cell and a culture medium for said hybrid.

The following claim is limited to the deposited cell line:

US 4,558,006
> As a new composition, a hybridoma cell line A.T.C.C. HB8209
> that produces a monoclonal antibody specifically
> immunoreactive with erythropoietin and with a polypeptide
> substantially duplicative of an amino acid sequence extant in
> erythropoietin.

In the few examples to be given of patents for the preparation of monoclonal antibodies the first is worthy of special mention. This patent was granted in the USA but the corresponding application in the UK was refused and the corresponding application in Japan, although allowed by the Patent Office, was opposed by a third party. It will be seen from the claim given below that the patent relates to the application of the basic Milstein/Kohler method to a particular class of antibodies, i.e. those which react to viruses.

US 4,196,265
> A process for producing viral antibodies comprising fusing a
> viral antibody producing cell and a myeloma cell to provide a
> fused cell hybrid, culturing said hybrid and collecting the viral
> antibodies.

In the UK the Patent Office took the view that since the basic monoclonal antibody technique had already been published it was obvious to apply this technology to an area where it had already been considered valuable, i.e. for viruses. The British Patent Office also would not allow a specific claim to the particular hybridoma developed for producing monoclonal antibodies against influenza virus. The applicant had not shown that the preparation of hybridomas of this type required anything other than the application of known techniques and moreover none of the hybridomas could be said to have particularly unusual advantages.

Nevertheless some broad patents are issuing in the UK as shown by the two following examples.

UK 2,115,005
> An anti-rat liver monoclonal antibody naturally capable of
> detecting an antigen associated with mammalian hepatocytes
> but not with normal syngenetic cell types.

UK 2,083,836
> (a broadly similar claim is present in US 4,423,147)
> A monoclonal antibody produced by a hybrid cell line

characterised in that the antibody has specificity to interferon-α.

Many claims for monoclonal antibodies are presented in terms of more detailed properties such as:

US 4,363,799

A monoclonal antibody of class IgG produced by a hybridoma formed by fusion of cells from a mouse myeloma line and spleen cells from a mouse previously immunised with human T cells, which antibody:

(a)   reacts with essentially all normal human peripheral T cells but not with normal human peripheral B cells, null cells or macrophages;

(b)   reacts with from about 5% to about 10% of normal human thymocytes;

(c)   reacts with leukemic cells from humans with T cell chronic lymphoblastic leukemia but does not react with leukemic cells from humans with T cell acute lymphoblastic leukemia;

(d)   exhibits a pattern of reactivity with the human T cell lines HDJ-1, CEM and HSB-2 shown in Figure 4; and

(e)   does not react with Epstein-Barr virus-transformed human B cell lines.

Finally, many patents are being granted based on the use of monoclonal antibodies and systems containing them in diagnostic assays. In these the claims are directed either to the method of assay or to particular reagent compositions or to combinations of materials useful in diagnostic kits. The single example given below is that of an important patent which has been the subject of litigation in the USA.

US 4,376,110

The invention lay in the use of monoclonal antibodies in place of prior art polyclonal antibodies in a known sandwich assay system. When the US Patent Office originally examined the application it argued that it would be obvious to use monoclonal antibodies in place of polyclonals in conventional immunoassay protocols. This objection was overcome by including in the claims a numerical limitation regarding the affinity (binding power) of the antibodies. In the District Court the patent was held invalid on the grounds of obviousness, as many would have predicted, but this was overruled by the Court of Appeals for the Federal Circuit.

Much of the case turned on aspects of US patent law relating to priority of invention which have no parallel in the patent laws of Europe and most other countries. Reference to laboratory notebooks and other evidence in order to determine priority of invention is crucial under the US first-to-invent system but is inadmissible under the European or any other first-to-file system of patent law (see Chapter 3, Question 23). But on the question of inventiveness the court upheld the patent because the prior art was 'devoid of any suggestion that monoclonal antibodies can be used in the same fashion as polyclonals'. Also, it was influenced by the commercial success of the patentee's product and found that a 3 year time gap between the first availability of monoclonals and the sale of the patentee's kits was long enough to indicate lack of obviousness. The court also gave short shrift to the 'obvious to try' argument.

The decision given in this case contrasts with that given by the British Patent Office, mentioned above, concerning the patent application for monoclonal antibodies to viruses. Although the subject matter was different in each case the fundamental issue is one of the inventiveness or obviousness of particular applications of a recently discovered general technique. It should be remembered that decisions given in contested cases depend very much on the specific circumstances and the way the inventions are presented to the courts. Although courts are sometimes helped by experts the problem of assessing complex technology and of making the difficult determination of inventiveness is acute.

8   Legal protection for plants and animals

The two previous chapters have concentrated on areas of central interest to the pharmaceutical and agrochemical industries and to those who work in these technologies in research institutions. Industrial firms which have entered the field of biotechnology have displayed in this area the same strong attachment to patent protection that they have shown for novel drugs and other chemical compounds. The biotechnology of plants and animals, however, impinges on agriculture and animal husbandry, two fields of endeavour in which attitudes to legal protection have traditionally been rather different. Until this impact can be better understood a certain tension may exist between those working in the different disciplines involved. Most of this chapter will be concerned with the legal protection of plants where legal systems may compete with one another in demonstrating relevance to certain kinds of innovation.

The protection of plants

Many of the processes being developed in plant biotechnology can be protected straightforwardly under the patent system provided they comply with the basic patentability criteria of novelty, inventiveness, and practical application. Thus plant cell and tissue culture methods and the use of plant cells, e.g. in immobilised or other form for the production of valuable chemical products, are considered by patent examining authorities to be within the general category of microbiological process inventions. These are accordingly patentable as processes. Up to a point, the new products of such processes may also be patented. These processes, in which plant cells are a means to an end, are recognised as industrial processes broadly comparable to the cultivation of micro-organisms for the preparation of other products such as antibiotics, enzymes and vitamins. Patenting in this area will be subject to the same constraints as affect other microbiological inventions and which are now clear from experience. Thus the deposition in official culture collections of novel strains and other essential biological material will apply here also and will raise again the debated question of the merits of patenting versus industrial or trade secrecy.

Where the object of the innovation is to produce a new or improved plant there is a potential impact on agriculture and horticulture which must be evaluated. In Europe and many other countries agricultural processes and products (but not agricultural equipment) were considered in the past to be outside the realm of the patent law. The European Patent Convention of 1973, however, declared agriculture to be on the same footing as other industries as regards the criterion of 'industrial applicability' which is necessary to establish the patentability of any invention under European law. Nevertheless Article 53(b) of the Convention states that European patents shall *not* be granted in respect of

> 'plant or animal varieties or essentially biological processes for the production of plants or animals; this provision does not apply to microbiological processes or the products thereof.'

This exclusion is said to be justified by the fact that new plant varieties are protectable under another system of law, namely, the Plant Variety Right to be discussed below. By contrast the United States, always the exception in any comparative description of patent law, has permitted patents to be granted on plant breeding methods and products as well as allowing protection for varieties under the other form of legal right known as the Certificate of Variety Protection.

Plant variety rights

The intention of the plant variety right system was to give to the breeder broadly similar incentives and opportunities for reward as were available to inventors under the patent system. However, because a plant is a self-reproducing mechanism which can give rise to an indefinite number of descendants and quantity of consumption material, the legislators deliberately restricted the scope of plant variety protection. Thus the line was drawn by reference to *propagation* and the *intention* of the propagator of the new variety. The activities covered by this form of right are limited to (a) the production for sale and (b) the sale of *reproductive* material with the intention that it be used *as such*, e.g. seed for sowing.

These rights are granted under national laws but there is also an International Convention governing them (UPOV) which was drawn up in 1961 and became effective in 1968. This states the nature of the right as covering:

> 'production for purposes of commercial marketing, offer for sale and marketing of the reproductive or vegetative propagating material as such.'

The right does not extent to the saving of seed from a current crop for sowing in a later season (the 'farmer's privilege'). Also it does not cover the production and sale of consumption material of the new variety, e.g. fruit or grain. Finally, the right does not prevent the use of the protected variety as source material for the addition of further variation in order to create yet another variety unless commercial production of the latter requires the repeated use of the protected variety (the 'research exemption'). For the traditional plant breeder and the farmer or grower it was considered necessary to preserve these freedoms.

The UPOV Convention also provides that any member state can provide patent protection or plant variety right protection, but not both, for the same botanical species or genus. Hence the exclusion of plant varieties from patent protection in Article 53(b) mentioned above.

The main difference between plant variety rights and patent rights is that the former gives no protection for enabling technology. Because the plant variety right protects only propagating material it does not cover process technology for the production of new varieties even where this is applicable to a wider range of plant materials than the individual variety of a particular species. Also the scope of protection for the new variety is limited much more by reference to the biological material itself than by reliance on a written specification. In seeking protection for a plant variety it is necessary for the breeder to supply an objective description of the new variety and to list its characteristics in a qualitative or quantitative way by means of which it is distinguished from previously known varieties. One can think of a plant variety therefore as a 'description' to which a particular plant must conform within a range of defined characteristics. These characteristics may be regarded as to some extent similar to the component parts of a patent claim but the comparison should not be pressed too far. In practice the owner of plant variety rights will most usually be exercising those rights against persons who have obtained the protected variety and are improperly dealing in it, i.e. the infringer's plants will have been derived by descent from the propagating material which was developed by the holder of the rights. It is also apparently possible, though rare, for two breeders working independently of one another to alight on the 'same' variety. In this case the first to apply for protection will prevail and will be able to prevent unauthorised use of the other's product. The test of infringement in such a case would presumably be by comparison of the plant materials and by reference to the defined characteristics of the protected variety.

Patents on plant genetic manipulation

Methods for the production of new plant types will be patentable as methods (processes) whether the approach is by the recombinant or non-recombinant route. The reagents and other tools of these methodologies will also be patentable including the development of new vector systems and gene inserts and methods of transforming cells. Transformed plant cells should also be patentable as products. In the non-recombinant field inventive processes based on the use of somaclonal variation technology, protoplast fusion, micropropagation and so on are open to patent protection because they are properly classified as microbiological methods or because they involve such a degree of human technical intervention that they cannot be classed as 'essentially biological' methods. Inventions which solve the problem of regenerating whole plants from transformed plant cells must also be patentable.

The primary difficulty posed by the present law in European countries is whether the final plants produced by any of these methods can be patented as products in the face of Article 53(b). The greater flexibility of the United States patent law in allowing new plants to be patented has been confirmed in a recent case on a maize seed having a specified minimum endogenous free tryptophan content achieved by tissue culture and selection techniques.

US 4,581,847

> To produce a maize seed having an unusually high content of free tryptophan the patentees set up a number of maize tissue cultures in the presence of inhibitory levels of a tryptophan analogue, e.g. 5-methyl tryptophan, in order to select a stable analogue resistant cell line from which maize plants could be regenerated. The patent mentions the fact that similar techniques had already been used for tobacco, carrot, potato and other cell lines. The main claim reads
>
> 'A maize seed having an endogenous free tryptophan content of at least about one-tenth milligram per gram dry seed weight and capable of germinating into a plant capable of producing seed having an endogenous free tryptophan content of at least about one-tenth milligram per gram dry seed weight.'

For such a patent to be allowed in Europe would be of major significance bearing in mind the official interpretation of Article 53(b) of the European Patent Convention. It would be possible to argue that such a claim was not a claim to a new variety. Alternatively the seed could be said to be the product of a microbiological process and therefore patentable under the second limb of Article 53(b). There is no real justification for this quirk of the patent law in Europe and it is desirable to have the situation clarified or the law changed.

> *The European Patent office have allowed a patent with a claim to*
>
> 'Propagating material for cultivated plants, treated with an oxime derivative according to formula I . . . '.
>
> *This claim was allowed after an appeal to the Technical Board of Appeals. The original objection that this claimed a plant variety was clearly misconceived but the Examiner no doubt felt in need of higher authority to allow such a claim in view of the possible application of Article 53(b). The Board held that this prohibited only the patenting of plants or their propagating material in the genetically fixed form of the plant variety, which was not the case here. Moreover the claimed propagating material was not the result of an essentially biological process for the breeding of plants but the result of treatment with a seed dressing agent to protect seeds against certain herbicides.*

The Swiss Patent Office has been the first to declare that patents will be allowed for new plants provided the claims are not directed to individual varieties, i.e. are more general in scope. This enlightened approach may now spread to other jurisdictions.

Patenting plant genes

Whatever the prospects for plant patents there will be no obstacle to the patenting of novel DNA sequences which give rise to useful properties when inserted into a plant chromosome or at some other site. In principle these patents should have the same legal effect as other patents for chemical compounds and should therefore extend to all compositions containing them and to all uses to which they are applied to exploit their properties. This view of the effect of such patents is a robust view of the situation. Genes are not very like industrial chemical compounds which when formulated into mixtures are usually fairly readily detectable in significant quantities. When new genetic material is inserted into a plant genome reliance may have to be placed on detecting the property for which the gene is responsible in order to prove that the plant is an infringing plant. There will be no shortage of difficult problems such as this to be faced by courts of law as the result of the progress of biotechnology.

The protection of animals

For novel animal breeders there is no system of legal protection comparable to the plant variety right. The justification for including animal varieties in Article 53(b) and its counterparts in certain national laws is therefore less obvious. Transgenic animals are now being developed by biotechnology and this will begin fairly soon to bring pressure on the patent law. In the United States the first animal test case has arisen. The US law has no exclusion corresponding to Article 53(b) of the European law but, as in the maize seed case, an appeal from the Examiner's rejection was necessary.

> *The claim in the Allen* et al. *application was to a polyploid Pacific oyster produced by a certain process of applying hydrostatic pressure to the zygotes. The Examiner had argued that the claim was to living matter controlled by laws of nature and not by man and hence unpatentable. But the Board held that the Chakrabarty case (see page 89) had established that the sole issue was whether the subject matter was man-made as distinct from occurring naturally. The Board refused the claim on other grounds but the importance of the case lies in their rejection of the Examiner's argument mentioned above.*

The idea of patents for animals has apparently raised in some minds the question of its extension to humans, surely one of the most bizarre applications of the *reductio ad absurdum* argument yet to be devised. But the rapid strides already made in biotechnology should condition us away from complacency and to face even this possibility. Since the abolition of slavery and other laws treating human beings as chattels there can be no property rights in humans. Patent law already excludes inventions contrary to '*ordre publique*' or morality. The patent law officials will simply require all patents conceivable in this field to be restricted to non-human animals but even apart from the natural conservatism which will operate against any such extravagant notions public policy will undoubtedly intervene if necessary to build such restrictions into the law.

9 Miscellaneous questions

After the more formal presentations given in the last three chapters we return now to the question and answer method of dealing briefly with certain topics that have been omitted so far. First is the question of financial benefit to an inventor. Secondly comes the question of infringement of a patent, a subject which would require a special chapter in a more formal textbook of patent law. Infringement is a matter of national patent law and there are variations of approach from country to country on this issue. Patent litigation is an expensive activity and decisions to proceed in the courts are invariably taken at high level in industrial companies. The individual research worker should however be aware of the basic principles because these have a definite bearing on the way patents are written.

1 How can I benefit financially from a patent?

This depends first upon whether you own the patent rights or whether these vest in your employer. This in turn depends upon whether the invention has arisen in the course of your normal research duties which you carry out on behalf of your employer or some other body which is funding the work. Most inventions that are patented arise from research carried out in industrial laboratories or elsewhere and ownership resides in the employer. The patent is usually taken out in the name of the employer but naming the inventors on the printed patent specification. US patents are granted to the inventors but an assignee employer may be recorded on the patent.

2 Should a contract of employment make reference to ownership of inventions?

A contract of service ought to deal with this question explicitly. Even if patents and other intellectual property rights are not mentioned in the terms of employment, however, it can usually be determined from consideration of the duties of the employee whether the invention belongs to him or the employer.

3 Is the position different in the case of non-commercial institutions devoted to research?

The situation here is somewhat less certain than in the case of an industrial establishment but the decisive test is whether the words of the statute apply to the particular research worker and to the invention. For example British patent law contains special sections devoted to employee inventions and the wording is not restricted to industrial employers and employees. The test is whether the invention has arisen in the course of the normal duties of the employee or duties specially assigned to him. However some universities, for example, might take the view that they are a community of scholars who have no duty to be innovators. In the absence of controlling case law it is better for a university to work out with its research staff a policy which is fair to all concerned. The abstract question of legal ownership is usually far less important than the question of responsibility for exploitation and the sharing of the resultant benefits.

4 But surely an inventor has a right to some compensation?

Not in the ordinary course of events because the individual may be paid to carry out research work or the status of the job may be such that original research is expected as part of the duties involved. British law does include provision for compensation of an inventor, even where ownership resides with the employer, but only where the patent is of outstanding benefit to the employer.

5 What is the position of the inventor in the case of contract research?

Where the research worker works in an academic or similar institution, or where he is employed in a commercial contract research organisation, the research contract should spell out the expectations of the sponsor and the invention-generating body. Where the sponsor is providing the bulk of the funds necessary to support the research the sponsor will usually claim absolute ownership of any rights or may claim the privilege of deciding how these rights will be apportioned or utilised. Research contracts will usually follow one or more of the set patterns but everything is negotiable. Research organisations should consider some provision for compensation of the inventors, or some extra benefit to themselves, beyond the funding of the work where the invention turns out to be of outstanding benefit to the sponsor.

6   Who owns a cell line – the human source of the original cells or the scientists who develop the cell line?

The cell line may be one established from the original cells without hybridisation and it may be useful as a host cell for culturing viruses or other materials. Alternatively it could be a hybridoma developed as a source of a particular antibody.

The question involves two kinds of property, the tangible kind (personal property) and the kind with which this book is concerned (intellectual property). There have been cases in which these issues have been involved especially in the USA. Most have been settled out of court because the issues are fraught with uncertainty. The settlements are usually based on a division of the benefit from manufacturing the cell line or from licensing the intellectual property. Patent law is especially amenable to mechanisms for distribution of rights or income. Usually the abstract question of ownership of the personal property, or even the intellectual property, can be side-stepped in favour of monetary settlements which are often of paramount importance in such disputes. The original donor of the cells which have been used to develop the cell line cannot claim to be an inventor under patent law since he or she will usually have had no conception of the potential of these cells and will have played no technical part in the development of a useful product.

7   If in the course of my research I discover that someone already holds a patent which is relevant to my work what should I do?

The first thing to have checked is whether the patent is still in force. It is possible that the patent may have lapsed at the end of its normal life or it may have been allowed to lapse at some earlier stage by non-payment of renewal fees. A great deal of abortive study and worry can be avoided if this simple precaution is taken. Only when the patent is found to be in force does one need to go further. Then might be the time to take professional advice especially if the legal scope of the patent is not crystal clear. It would be foolish to draw important conclusions without proper advice.

8   Presumably someone else's patent need only concern me if I am intending to use the invention commercially?

A word of caution is necessary here. If the patent is for a piece of laboratory equipment, for example, it might not always follow that one is free to make up one's own version of this equipment for use in the laboratory simply on the ground that there is no sale of any product. In

UK law there are certain acts which are exempted from being infringements and these include acts

(a) done privately and for purposes which are not commercial, or

(b) done for experimental purposes relating to the subject matter of the invention.

In this respect the British law is harmonised with the Community Patent Convention, i.e. a patent system for the member states of the European Economic Community ('Common Market').

9 Is infringement decided solely by the wording of the patent claims?

The wording of the claims is of the greatest importance. If the product or process which is said to infringe falls clearly within the words of the claim there will be no doubt about infringement. Of course, in order to be infringed, the claims must be valid. This means that if there is any serious prior art which throws doubt on the validity of the claims, or which requires them to be construed in a somewhat limited way in order to avoid the prior art, an infringement action might not succeed in court. In some countries there is a doctrine of 'equivalents' which can be invoked by the patentee where the defendant is not operating within the strict terms of the claims. According to European patent law the true scope of the claims must be decided by reference to the language of the claims but also by the specification as a whole; this is not so much a question of equivalents but of the proper interpretation of the scope of a claim. The literal wording of the claim therefore does not finally dispose of the matter. US law also has the doctrine of equivalents which can in suitable cases be relied upon where the alleged infringing product performs 'substantially the same function in substantially the same way to yield substantially the same result' as the patented product. One other important way in which a patent can be infringed without directly making or doing something covered by the claims is to produce a product or to perform an act which induces a third party to complete the act of infringement. This is commonly described as contributory infringement.

10 Can an example be given to illustrate the previous answer?

A recent example concerns the patent on the selective herbicide glyphosate which has been the subject of litigation in UK and other countries. Glyphosate (phosphonomethyl glycine) was a known compound at the time its herbicidal properties were discovered and so the first claim of the UK Patent 1,366,379 is directed to herbicidal compositions containing glyphosate or certain novel derivatives of glyphosate as active ingredients. Among these derivatives listed in the claim is a group of salts of the acid defined by reference to specific cation components, e.g. alkali metal, ammonium, organic ammonium. The defendants marketed formulations based on a glyphosate salt which was not listed in the patent claim, namely, the trimethylsulphonium salt. The patentee (plaintiff) alleged that glyphosate salts in the aqueous solutions typically used to apply the herbicide are ionised and that the active 'killer' component is in fact the anion of glyphosate or the glyphosate derivative. The patent also contains a specific claim to aqueous solutions of glyphosate. The plaintiff argued that the glyphosate anion was common to all glyphosate salts including the defendants' salt and was therefore the essential part of the claim for purposes of determining the scope of the patent. The defendants' counter-argument was that the patentee had limited the claim by a precise chemical definition which did not include the salt marketed by them and therefore could not now be extended by some theory of biological action. Furthermore, the defendants argued that at the time of publication of the patent the skilled reader would have no idea how these compositions acted to kill undesired plants.

The final resolution of this issue in various countries has not yet been determined.

11   How is indirect or contributory infringement to be understood?

United States law has been the first to deal explicity with this matter. It provides that:

> '. . . whoever without authority makes, uses or sells any patented invention within the United States . . . infringes the patent' (direct infringement)

but also

> 'whoever actively induces infringement of the patent shall be liable as an infringer' (inducement to infringe)

and

> 'whoever sells a component part of a patented machine, manufacture, combination or composition, or a material or apparatus for use in practicing a patented process constituting a material part of the invention, knowing the same to be especially made or especially adapted for use in an infringement of such patent, and not a staple article or commodity of commerce suitable for substantial non-infringing use, shall be liable as a contributory infringer' (contributory infringement).

The contributory infringement provision has been applied by the Supreme Court to prevent the sale of propanil as a herbicide for use in a patented method of treatment of rice crops. The compound itself could not be patented but its herbicidal use was.

United Kingdom law now spells out the various acts which constitute infringement of product patents and process patents. It also includes a contributory infringement provision covering the supply of any of the means, relating to an essential element of the invention, for putting the invention into effect, provided this is done in the knowledge of the intended use of such means. In conformity with European law, UK patent law provides that a process patent gives protection for any product obtained directly by the process.

12   Does experimental use count as infringement?

The question of experimental use can arise in two different ways. The first of these has been touched on in Chapter 3 in answer to Questions 21 and 22 (pp. 33, 34). This dealt with the extent to which an inventor's own use of his invention prior to filing a patent application was permitted as experimental use rather than being a prior use which would invalidate the patent. For the present question we are mainly concerned with experimental use by others, after a patent has been granted, and whether such use would be an infringement of the patent. Nevertheless if an experimental use defence is raised in an infringement action the court has to determine whether the particular use which is claimed as permissible is in fact experimental as understood from previous case law. Just such an issue arose in the infringement action on the glyphosate patent mentioned in answer to Question 10. To deal with it the British Court reviewed case law over a long period going back as far as 1844, much of which was concerned with the invalidatory aspect of prior use mentioned at the beginning of this answer.

> In the glyphosate case, the question was whether the defendants'
> field trials of their compound was permitted experimental use.
> There were three categories of field trial:
> 1.   On the defendants own farm.
> 2.   On rented land on other farms.
> 3.   On publicly owned land by agricultural and other public
>   bodies as required by official regulatory approval
>   procedures.
> Only the first of these was allowed by the British Court of Appeal
> as 'acts done for experimental purposes relating to the subject
> matter of the patented invention'. The Court held that trials
> carried out to discover something unknown or to test a hypothesis
> or to see if something will work under different conditions, can
> be fairly regarded as experiments, but trials carried out to
> demonstrate something to a potential customer or other body for

purposes of approval of a product, could not be so regarded. Among the precedents cited in this case was a decision of the Supreme Court of Canada in which the test-manufacture of a small quantity of a patented drug (trifluoroperazine) by a company which had applied for a compulsory licence under the patent was held to be experimental. Such use was not for profit but to establish that the potential licensee could make the product in accordance with the specification.

In the United States there have been a fair number of cases on this issue. There is a line of cases in which the experimental use defence has been allowed and another line in which it has been refused. The guiding principles appear to have been laid down in two cases decided in 1813 and current US professional opinion believes that these principles are valid today. An experiment 'to ascertain the veracity and exactness of the specification' or one carried out as a 'philosophical experiment' will not be an infringement but it must also be clear that the experiment is not carried out with the 'intent to use for profit'.

It can probably be concluded that European and United States patent law take much the same view of experimental use. Experimental use *on* patented inventions must be distinguished from using patented inventions *for* experimental purposes. This is probably what is intended by the British Statute and the Community Patent Convention which state that the experiment must relate to the subject matter of the invention. It is quite clear therefore that it will be no defence simply to say that the invention is being used in a research laboratory. However there will always be room for argument on this question. One area which still remains rather grey is where the experiment is designed to improve upon a particular invention and where the improvement constitutes a further invention which is outside the claims of the patent on the original invention. Most people would tend to regard this as fair game between competitive research groups.

13   Are there any special problems involved in stopping the infringement of biotechnology patents?

If the patent is for a product which will be put on the market there should be no special problem beyond the usual necessity to show that the product falls within the scope of the patent claims. This may be apparent from an inspection or analysis of the product concerned and, assuming that the product claims are of the strongest type, i.e. *per se* claims, it would usually be unnecessary to show how the product was made. Where the patent is for a process, or the product claims are those of the product-by-process type, there will often be the problem of providing proof of infringement, that is, showing that the patented process has been used to make the final marketed product. Problems of this sort are common to process patents of many kinds, also in chemistry and even in non-chemical processes,where it is difficult or impossible to tell from an examination of the product what process has been used to make it. In biotechnology this difficulty may be enhanced by the variability of living matter which offers more scope for argument over the identity of biological systems and the derivation of one from another.

For biotechnology patents which depend upon a defined micro-organism a further problem arises from the relative ease with which micro-organisms can be modified, either by conventional mutagenic treatment or by direct chemical treatment of DNA molecules. These present the applicant with substantial problems of proof of derivation from the deposited strain. In any case the legal question of patent infringement by modification of deposited organisms is by no means clear and settled. The question of derivation, for example, must be decided by expert scientific evidence, which may be conflicting. In one British case on a patent for a process for producing tetracycline, there was contradictory evidence upon whether the strain used by the defendants was a *Streptomyces aureofaciens* of the kind claimed in the patent, or whether it could have been derived by mutation of a micro-organism which, both sides agreed, was not of this species.

An account of this case is given as case study 3 in Chapter 10.

14   **How then can one stop an infringing process when it is carried out under commercial secrecy?**

This is a problem to which patent law cannot give a totally satisfying answer. The general problem is obviously not unique to patent law and many other laws are broken by the unscrupulous in the hope that such breaches will not be discovered. The enforcement of a law requires a mechanism for discovery of the offence and this involves the difficult question of intrusion into the affairs and premises of others who may in fact be innocent after all. The discovery of patent infringement in these circumstances has to fall under the rules of procedure and evidence which obtain under the general legal system of any country.

The position of the patentee is not hopeless however and there are some established principles which can help him. As a rule the burden of proof lies with the complainant but in the laws of many countries this burden can be reversed if a *prima facie* case of infringement can be made out or in other circumstances. Where the product is a new product the law of some countries states that it will be assumed that the product made by the alleged infringer will have been made by the patented process unless evidence is shown to the contrary. This is known as a provision of 'reversal of the burden of proof'. Of course if the patent has a claim to the product there will be no need to rely on this provision but there may be cases in which for some reason only a process claim or a product-by-process claim can be obtained. Sometimes a chemical analysis of the product will show traces of substances used in the process of manufacture and this may give an indication helpful to proving infringement. One striking example of this, in a non-biological context, is the well known float glass process of making plate glass with excellent surface finish by passing a layer of the molten glass over the surface of a bath of molten tin instead of grinding and polishing the surface of the glass by the prior art method. When the float glass method is used traces of tin will be found in the surface of the product. Another use of the *prima facie* case is where it can be shown that no way of making a particular product is known other than by the patented process. If the product is produced by a micro-organism and it can be shown that the competing manufacturer has obtained the patentee's strain from the culture collection in which it has been deposited for patent purposes this could be helpful towards making out a *prima facie* case. It is of course not conclusive because competitors are allowed access to deposited micro-organisms for legitimate purposes of evaluation and it does not follow that they are using the deposited strain commercially.

The difficulty of 'policing' patents which do not claim a marketed product has to be faced at the outset when one is deciding whether to patent or not to patent. More discussion of this issue is given in Appendix 3.

15   Does a patent protect against importation of a product?

Provided a patent has suitable claims to cover the product it can prevent importation of the product just as effectively as if the product had been manufactured locally. Where the patent is for a process its power to prevent importation of a product made by the process in another country, e.g. where no corresponding patent has been taken out, will depend on the relevant law. In many countries the process patent extends to protect the product of the process. At present the USA is one exception to this but there have been proposals to introduce a law which will extend the scope of a process patent in this respect. There is optimism that such a law will soon be passed in the USA. It will be realised that obtaining proof that the patented process has been used abroad may be difficult for the patentee to obtain because the power of the court in which he is suing for infringement is limited to its own national jurisdiction.

10　Case studies

Many of the points dealt with in the question and answer sections and elsewhere in this book can be seen in a practical setting in the following brief summaries of actual case histories. When a patent situation is in process of development an applicant usually prefers to keep his own counsel as regards tactics and to minimise the amount of information that hostile competitors might acquire and possibly exploit to his disadvantage. Much information can be gleaned from an examination of Patent Office files when these are or become available to the public. But case studies can be most openly discussed when the case is over and done with or reaching the end of its period of legal protection. The first two which follow are of this kind.

Case study 1: enzyme anticoagulant

This first case study relates to the patenting of an enzyme extracted from snake venom and of interest in anticoagulant therapy.

A team of research workers at a Malayan research institute had submitted a paper for publication in *The Lancet* in 1963 describing the effects of snake bite from the Malayan pit viper (*Ancistrodon Rhodostoma*). It was found that the patient's blood was rendered incoagulable for many days after a bite and that during this time there were no episodes of severe bleeding. This anticoagulant effect appeared to be the result of conversion of circulating fibrinogen to fibrin in a harmless form. These results had suggested to the authors that a suitable venom fraction might have therapeutic application and they had made this suggestion in the text of the paper first submitted to the journal. At this stage they took advice on patenting and were advised that no effective protection could be obtained until they had developed a fractionation procedure and could at least partly identify the active component.

Whilst the paper was being processed by the journal the two main authors, knowing that interest would be shown by industry on publication of their work, subjected the venom to precipitation with methanol as the first step of a possible fractionation method. With limited facilities, it was not possible to take purification much further in the time remaining before the expected publication date and it was too late to withdraw the paper. It was then decided that a patent application should be filed protecting the work as so far developed although it was realised that nothing might come of it in the absence of further purification along the lines they would suggest in a preliminary specification. Only these two of the co-authors were considered to be inventors. Although the authors were unwilling to suspend publication until they had isolated the active component they agreed to remove from the text all reference to possible therapeutic application, on the advice of their patent agent.

The two original inventors were unable to complete the purification and identification of the important component without bringing in a co-worker having expertise in the fractionation of venoms. A different method of purification was now followed and this was successful in isolating the desired enzyme in pure form for characterisation. It was considered, therefore, that the preliminary application should be abandoned in favour of a fresh application naming three co-inventors and based on the perfected purification procedure using column chromatography.

The new patent application resulted in the grant of UK Patent 1,094,301, the text of which is reproduced in Figs. 10.1–10.4. An equivalent US Patent No. 3,657,416, and corresponding patents in other countries were also obtained.

In this case it was vital to obtain good product claims, as it was by no means certain that the chromatographic purification procedure described by way of example in the patent would be the process adopted by an industrial licensee for use on a commercial scale. There was no better way known at the time of characterising an enzyme of the molecular size involved than by the combination of physical, chemical, and biological data included in the main product claim. In any case this was the best information that the inventors could provide. The enzyme came to be called 'Arvin' (generic name Ancrod).

The US patent application

The United States Examiner first objected that the product was not properly defined and referred to the data as 'a few arbitrary characteristics'. The Examiner also objected that, being a product of nature, the enzyme was not patentable. An additional objection was that no evidence of biological utility had been provided.

The question whether the product had been adequately characterised continued to be a disputed point throughout the prosecution of the application. It was argued that the inventors had given their best evidence which was scientifically accurate and acceptable and this was finally accepted, although reluctantly. The 'product of nature' objection was short lived because it gave way to a lack of novelty objection based

PATENT SPECIFICATION

NO DRAWINGS

Inventors: HUGH ALISTAIR REID, KOK EWE CHAN and MICHAEL PETER ESNOUF

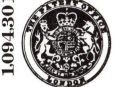

1,094,301

Date of filing Complete Specification: Feb. 19, 1965.

Application Date: Feb. 21, 1964.   No. 7264/64.

Complete Specification Published: Dec. 6, 1967.

© Crown Copyright 1967.

Index at acceptance: —**A5** B(2Z, 12A); **C3** H3

Int. Cl.: —**A 61 k 3/52**

COMPLETE SPECIFICATION

Improvements relating to Anticoagulants

We, NATIONAL RESEARCH DEVELOPMENT CORPORATION, a British Corporation, established by Statute, of Kingsgate House, 66—74 Victoria Street, London, S.W.1, do hereby declare the invention, for which we pray that a patent may be granted to us, and the method by which it is to be performed, to be particularly described in and by the following statement:—

This invention is concerned with substances having activity in relation to the clotting of mammalian blood.

The clotting of human and other mammalian blood proceeds by a complicated mechanism which occurs in distinct stages. In the last stage of the process blood fibrinogen is converted by means of the enzyme thrombin into "fibrin monomer" which then undergoes polymerisation to produce fibrin, the material of the clot. It has now been discovered that there exists in the venom of *Ancistrodon Rhodostoma* (*Boie*) (the Malayan pit viper) an enzyme which has a thrombin-like action but which modifies bloor fibrinogen in such a way that the fibrin produced from it has different properties from those of the normal thrombin-formed clot. Fibrin induced by this enzyme is of a wispy character and as a result of the continual flow of blood in vivo it is insensibly dispersed in the blood passages so that clot formation does not occur. It has been found that *A. Rhodostoma* venom may be purified by removal of proteolytic constituents which cause severe local reaction and other undesirable side effects to produce a purified fraction of the venom in which the properties of the defibrinating anticoagulant enzyme may be utilised in therapy as well as for research purposes. It has more over been established that the active principle may be isolated from the venom

in highly pure form as hereinbefore described.

The purified active substance of this invention is characterised by the following physico-chemical and biological properties as determined on material containing not more than 1 or 2% protein impurity.

1. it is proteinaceous and substantially colourless when pure

2. it is adsorbed by weakly basic anion exchange material such as diethylaminomethyl cellulose and triethylaminoethyl cellulose

3. it is soluble in physiological saline

4. it has an electrophoretic mobility* of 3.9×10^{-5} volts/cm/sec. in 0.1M phosphate buffer pH 7.0,

5. it has a molecular weight not greater than 40,000 in monomeric form, as determined in the ultracentrifuge

6. it has a sedimentation co-efficient $S_{20}W = 3.4$ svedbergs at a concentration of 4.86 mg/ml.

7. it has a partial specific volume of 0.7 approximately, at a concentration of 4.86 mg/ml.

2. its biological activity is thrombin-like, and anticoagulant in vivo

9. it is not significantly inhibited by 1×10^{-3} molar di-isipropylfluorophosphate within 5 minutes.

*This figure is quoted in preference to the value of between 5.5 and 6.0 as determined in barbitrurate buffer at pH 8.6.

The active substance exerts its defibrinating effect rapidly after administration and persists in the body for long periods, e.g. up to two weeks in contrast to the heparin group of anticoagulants. On the other hand its action may be rapidly reversed by means of specific activenine. It is non-toxic, highly active at very low concentrations, and gives

[*Price 4s. 6d.*]

Fig. 10.1. Reproduced by kind permission of the Controller, H.M. Stationery Office.

rise to no spontaneous haemorrhagic complications.

It is highly specific in its action and appears to have no effect on other factors of the blood clotting mechanism than fibrinogen. As a result of this combination of properties it is valuable in the treatment of thrombosis, especially during the period in which the probability of a second and perhaps fatal attack is high. The pure substance is stable for very long periods at −20° C.

In accordance with the invention, a material useful in pharmaceutical preparations for the treatment of mammalian blood by parenteral administration is obtained by subjecting *A. Rhodostoma* venom to chromatography on weakly basic anion exchange suitable for adsorption of protein i.e. of sufficiently weak basicity to avoid denaturation of protein, and recovering from the material a fraction containing the active principle characterised above and substantially free of proteolytic enzymes which cause vascular and tissue necrosis. Suitable weakly basic anion exchange materials are certain polysaccharide materials containing tertiary amino (dialkylamino alkyl) groups and in practice DEAE-cellulose and TEAE-cellulose are highly convenient materials to use for the purpose of this invention, the latter being especially preferred on account of the greater ease with which it enables the active material to be separated from amino acid oxydase. The basic strength of the material, which is determined by the degree of substitution with the aminoethyl groups, is an important factor in preserving the stability of the active protein and should not be too high. The basicity of the material, usually expressed as milli-equivalents per gram, will in part determine the molarities of the eluting buffers employed in the separation, and optimum combinations will readily be settled by experiment. DEAE-"Sephadex" (Trade Mark) and similar materials have different basicities from DEAE-cellulose and will require the choice of appropriate buffer systems and concentrations.

The active material is recovered by elution of the anion exchange column and with DEAE-and TEAE-cellulose columns stepwise elution with buffers of increasing molarity, e.g. tris/phosphate buffer has given excellent results. This is an abbreviation of tris(hydroxymethyl)—amino methane. For example, with TEAE-cellulose of capacity 0.7 milli-equivalents/gram the undesirable constituents of the venom are eluted with tris/phosphate buffer at pH 6.0 in concentrations increasing step-wise up to about 0.04 M after which the active material may be eluted with the same buffer at concentrations from 0.09 M to 0.1 M or slightly higher. The solution of active material leaving the column may, if desired, be freeze-dried

to produce a light powder which may be stored in ampoules at low temperature either in bulk or in unit doses. Alternatively the solution may be made isotonic with normal physiological saline by the adjustment of its electrolytes with tris/phosphate or other buffer after which it may be sterilised e.g. by filtration to produce a composition usable directly for parenteral administration. This solution or one obtained by reconstitution of the freeze-dried powder may be given either intravenously or intramuscularly at a dosage of, for example 0.2—10 micrograms of active substance per kilo i.e. in dosage units of 14 to 700 micrograms. In the dog, dosages even as high as 1500 micrograms per kilo are tolerated without adverse effect and the blood is rendered incoagulable for long periods.

The invention is described in more detail in the following examples:

EXAMPLE 1

Triethylaminoethyl cellulose powder (Serva) of capacity 0.71 m.equiv./gm. is suspended in 2M sodium chloride buffered with 0.1 M tris/phosphate pH 6.0 and the slurry is packed into a glass column 3.6 cm. in diameter until the height of the packed material reaches 20 cm. The column is washed with a further 2L of the solvent used for preparing the slurry and is then equilibrated with 0.01 M tris/phosphate buffer pH 8.5. This is an abbreviation for tris-(hydroxymethyl)aminomethane.

330—360 mg. of crude *A. Rhodostoma* venom is dissolved in 20 ml. of 0.01 M tris/phosphate buffer pH 8.5, centrifuged to remove insoluble material, and the clear supernatant is applied to the column. The fractionation is carried out at room temperature at a flow rate of 90—100 ml./hour. The protein concentration in the eluate is estimated from the extinction of the solution at 280 mμ in 1 cm cells.

The chromatogram is developed with the following buffers. In all cases the molarity of the buffers are with respect to tris.

0.01 M tris/phosphate pH 8.5 (to wash venom onto the column) (fractions 1, 2, 3).
0.01 M tris/phosphate pH 7.0 (fraction 4)
0.02 M tris/phosphate pH 6.0—
0.04 M tris/phosphate pH 6.0 (fraction 5)
0.10 M tris/phosphate pH 6.0 (fraction 6)
0.10 M tris/phosphate+0.10 M NaCl pH 6.0 (fraction 7)

The changes in eluting buffer are made after the column has equilibrated with the buffer. The protein fractions obtained in this way are assayed for coagulant activity.

Less than 1% of the applied coagulant activity is recovered in fraction Nos. 1, 2, 3, 4. Fraction 1 however possesses proteolytic activity which in concentrated solutions would dissolve fibrin clots. The appearance of the

Fig. 10.2. Reproduced by kind permission of the Controller, H.M. Stationery Office.

1,094,301   3

coagulant activity is summarised in the following table.

Fraction No.	units/ml.	E_{280}	Specific Activity
Crude venom	100	0.174	574
5	9	0.085	106
6	78	0.0125	6240
7	35	0.0540	648

Units. these are arbitrary units, 100 units referring to the clotting time of the starting venom diluted (1/100)

E_{280} extinction of fraction at the dilution used for assay of the thrombin-like activity

The recovery of the thrombin-like material ranges between 50—65% in fraction 6, the remaining material appearing in fractions 5 and 7.

The thrombin-like activity is eluted from these columns in significant amounts at a buffer strength of 0.04 M or greater.

The eluate is freeze dried to give a light powdery product. Yield: 18—20 mg. per 350 mg. dry venom.

EXAMPLE 2

The procedure described in Example 1 takes about 36 hours to complete. A modification of the fractionation procedure, taking 14 hours, is as follows:

The length of the column is reduced to 15 cm. and equilibrated with 0.01 M tris/phosphate pH 6.0. The crude venom (350 mg.) is dissolved in 20 ml. 0.01 M tris/phosphate pH 6.0 and after centrifuging is applied to the column. The column is eluted with this buffer until no further protein is eluted, and then with the following:—

0.02 M tris/phosphate pH 6.0
0.035 M tris/phosphate pH 6.0
0.09 M tris/phosphate pH 6.0

The purity of the material obtained with this last-mentioned solvent is as good as obtained in Example 1, and, in some cases, the yield is increased to nearly 70%.

As in Example 1, the product may be recovered in freeze-dried form or the final solution may be adjusted to physiological pH and made isotonic by the addition of tris/phosphate and then sterilised by filtration.

Method of Assay of thrombin like activity 0.1 ml. oxalated bovine plasma is incubated at 37° C with 0.1 ml. 0.15 M sodium chloride buffered with 0.01 M tri-hydroxymethyl-amino-methane (tris)/Cl⁻ pH 7.5. To this is added 0.1 ml. 0.025 M $CaCl_2$ followed by 0.1 ml. of a fraction of the venom, and the clotting time of the mixture recorded. The clotting times obtained for a range of venom concentrations is plotted on log-log co-ordinates and a straight line is obtained.

In operating the process of extraction of the active material by chromatography on DEAE- or TEAE-cellulose, the pH, polarity, and other conditions are inter-related and best determined by experiment. As a guide, however, it may be stated that after elution of the proteolytic fraction the desired material may be eluted with tris/phosphate buffer in the pH range 5.5—7.5 and molarity of 0.04 M upwards, the total molarity of the solution being adjusted to at least 0.08, where necessary, with sodium chloride or other suitable salt.

WHAT WE CLAIM IS:—

1. An anticoagulant enzyme derivable from the venom of *Ancistrodon Rhodostoma* and characterised by the following properties:
   (1) it is proteinaceous and substantially colourless when pure
   (2) it is adsorbable on weakly basic anion exchange materials such as diethyl-aminoethyl cellulose and triethylamino-ethyl cellulose
   (3) it is soluble in physiological saline
   (4) it has an electrophoretic mobility of 3.9×10^{-5} volts/cm/sec. in 0.1 M phosphate buffer pH 7.0
   (5) it has a molecular weight not greater than 40,000 in monomeric form, as determined in the ultracentrifuge
   (6) it has a sedimentation co-efficient $S_{20}W=3.4$ svedbergs at a concentration of 4.86 mg/ml.
   (7) it has a partial specific volume of 0.7 approximately at a concentration of 4.86 mg/ml.
   (8) its biological activity is thrombin-like and anticoagulant in vivo.
   (9) it is not significantly inhibited by 1×10^{-3} molar diisopropylfluorophosphate within 5 minutes.

2. A pharmaceutical anticoagulant preparation comprising the enzyme defined in Claim 1 as the active constituent.

3. A pharmaceutical defibrinating sterile composition comprising the enzyme defined in Claim 1 dissolved in an aqueous medium and suitable for parenteral administration.

4. A pharmaceutical composition as defined in Claim 3 in which the aqueous medium comprises tris/phosphate buffer.

5. A pharmaceutical preparation as defined in Claim 2, comprising purified *Ancistrodon Rhodostoma* venom substantially free of proteolytic enzymes which cause tissue and vascular necrosis.

6. A pharmaceutical preparation as defined in Claim 2 comprising dosage unit of from 14 to 700 micrograms of active constituent.

7. A purified fraction of *Ancistrodon Rhodostoma* venom derived by chromtographic fractionation, having thrombin-like defibrinating properties, and substantially free from constituents of the venom which cause tissue and vascular necrosis.

8. Process for the preparation of an anti-

Fig. 10.3. Reproduced by kind permission of the Controller, H.M. Stationery Office.

4   1,094,301

coagulant material which comprises adsorbing *Ancistrodon Rhodostoma* venom on weakly basic anion exchange material suitable for adsorption of protein and recovering therefrom a fraction having thrombin-like defibrinating activity and substantially free from proteolytic enzymes which cause tissues and vascular necrosis.

9. Process according to Claim 8, in which the anion exchange material is a poly-saccharide containing dialkylaminoalkyl groups.

10. Process according to Claim 9, in which the anion exchange material is diethylamino-ethylcellulose or triethylaminoethyl cellulose.

11. Process according to Claim 10, in which a column of the anion exchange material is eluted in step-wise manner with tris/phosphate buffer of increasing molarity, the active fraction being collected after the said proteolytic constituents of the venom have been eluted.

12. Process according to Claim 11, in which the proteolytic and other unwanted constituents are eluted at pH 6 with buffer up to about 0.04 molar, the anticoagulant fraction being eluted with buffer of molarity 0.09—0.10.

13. Process according to any of Claims 8 to 12, in which the fraction recovered containing the anticoagulant material is freeze-dried.

14. Process according to Claim 11 or 12, in which the eluate containing the anti-coagulant material is rendered isotonic with normal physiological saline and sterilised.

15. Process according to Claim 11, substantially as described in Example 1.

16. Process according to Claim 11, substantially as described in Example 2.

17. Anticoagulant material when produced by a process according to any of the preceding Claims.

R. S. CRESPI,
Chartered Patent Agent,
Agent for the Applicants.

Leamington Spa: Printed for Her Majesty's Stationery Office by the Courier Press.—1967.
Published at The Patent Office, 25, Southampton Buildings, London, W.C.2, from which copies may be obtained.

ERRATA

SPECIFICATION No. 1,094,301

Page 1, line 24, *for* "bloor" *read* "blood"
Page 1, line 33, *for* "if" *read* "of"
Page 1, line 81, *for* "activenine" *read* "anti-venine"
Page 2, line 17, *after* "exchange" *insert* "material"
Page 2, line 54, *for* "This" *read* "Tris"
Page 2, line 98, *for* "This" *read* "Tris"
Page 3, line 48, *for* "isotomic" *read* "isotonic"
Page 4, line 8, *for* "tissues" *read* "tissue"

THE PATENT OFFICE
22 January 1968

Fig. 10.4. Reproduced by kind permission of the Controller, H.M. Stationery Office.

on a prior art reference to be mentioned later. In response to the lack of utility objection an affidavit was sworn by a medical practitioner who had investigated the clinical use of Arvin and had presented evidence to the British Dunlop Committee on the safety of drugs. The results of treatment of 13 patients were reported showing that the substance 'would appear to be a useful anticoagulant in certain clinical states'. The Examiner noted this rather indefinite statement made with the usual scientific caution. However the affidavit also said that the results 'showed convincingly that Arvin is successful in defibrinating the patient and therefore is likely to prevent the formation of a further clot . . . '.

The Examiner then cited a prior published paper by French workers on the separation of fractions of the same venom by electrophoresis. The Examiner's inference was that the prior workers must have isolated the same enzyme and had disclosed its properties. Analysis of the prior paper showed that the fractions isolated by the earlier workers were impure, had different properties altogether, and were of no therapeutic potential. Therefore the prior workers had not made the important finding of the presence of a defibrinating enzyme. Eventually this point was established by the repetition of the published experiments. This was carried out separately by two independent scientific experts, one in Britain and one in the USA, who attempted to reproduce as far as possible the apparatus and conditions described in the cited reference. These experiments failed to reveal the presence of a component having defibrinating properties in any of the fractions separated. Moreover none of these fractions possessed any useful therapeutic activity (rather the reverse) and the earlier work was not carried out with any intention of producing a useful product. The need to carry out experiments of this kind is a fairly common feature of US patent practice where it is necessary to show differences from what appears to be close prior art and also to show non-obviousness. The evidence is best produced from independent scientists and can now be made by way of declaration rather than affidavit.

The case for allowing the patent based on the above data and evidence was therefore cumulatively rather strong but it was still necessary to settle the matter by personal interview with Examiners in the US Patent Office requiring the attendance of the US attorney, the British patent agent, and one of the scientific experts.

The German patent application

German patent law did not allow product claims at the time the application was filed. Therefore the claims were drafted in terms of a process for preparing anticoagulant material from the venom based on chromatography on weakly basic anion exchange material. While the application was still pending, however, the German law changed and it became possible to introduce product claims. Consequently product claims based on the British model were added to the case.

The German Examiner cited as prior art a medical publication reporting on the properties of a commercial product known as 'Reptilase'. This was an extract of the venom of *Bothrops atrox* recommended as a haemostatic agent to stop blood flowing from wounds. The Examiner considered this prior product to be relevant and called for proof of the superiority of Arvin. The Examiner argued that in addition to having a haemostatic effect the prior product possessed anticoagulant activity and he therefore insisted on the furnishing of proof showing technical advance by comparison of the invention with the cited product.

The requirement to show technical advance over prior art no longer applies under German law but comparative tests can often be required and can be useful in demonstrating inventiveness over prior art.

It appeared to be difficult to set up proper comparative tests when the primary activity of the two substances being compared was of opposite character. Reptilase was a coagulant for use in conjunction with surgery whereas Arvin was anticoagulant and would not be used at the same time as surgery. Deadlock was reached with the Examiner on this point and in order to break it one of the inventors suggested a lateral approach showing the action on fibrinogen in plasma of the respective enzymes. In addition the inventor included tests on thrombin, the natural enzyme in blood which is involved in the clotting mechanism. Comparative blood clotting experiments were carried out using thrombin, Reptilase, and Arvin and the properties of the resulting fibrin clots were examined by the use of published methods. Under the action of thrombin, and later of factor VIII, the natural clot is a dense highly cross-linked structure containing a component known as alpha polymer. Reptilase also has an action on factor VIII. The Reptilase-induced clot also showed a significant alpha polymer component. By contrast Arvin has no action on factor VIII and the resulting micro clots contain no alpha polymer and are much more readily disposed of in the bloodstream. Thus by removing fibrinogen harmlessly from the system Arvin removes the material from which any subsequent thrombin-induced clot could be formed. The Examiner accepted this evidence as demonstrating superiority over Reptilase.

The Examiner then criticised the data used to characterise the enzyme in the product claim. Eventually by explaining in detail how these properties were determined and the fact that they were reliable parameters the Examiner accepted the claims. However this was not achieved without an interview at which the inventor who had provided much of the technical information was present to convince the Examiner on these points.

The enzyme patented in this case was claimed as derived from or derivable from the venom of *A. rhodostoma*. This was an acceptable limitation because the venom proved to be the only source, and a suitable one, for the purposes of commercial production of the anticoagulant. A limitation of this kind would require very careful consideration where a genetic engineering approach to its preparation could be contemplated.

Case study 2: poultry vaccine

This second case study concerns the development of a patent situation on a virus vaccine for protecting poultry against Marek's disease.

Workers at a British Poultry Research Institute had succeeded in isolating the causative agent of Marek's disease (MD) and had published this work in the journal '*Nature*' in 1967. The causative agent, which was considered to be a virus or a virus-like agent of the herpes group, had been isolated from chicken kidney cell monolayers inoculated with kidney cells from diseased birds. This publication occurred without consideration of patent possibilities. Later, some thought was given to the possible effect of this publication on the subsequent patenting of a vaccine should one be developed.

In the following year one of the original authors of the *Nature* publication discovered that important changes in the virus took place on passage in cell culture including the loss of certain antigens and a change in pathogenicity. These findings were described orally at the first International Congress for Virology in Helsinki in July 1968. This disclosure did not describe in full experimental detail the method used for attenuation of the virus and did not mention the fact that the attenuated virus was immunogenic. Also, the virulent strain of virus used as the starting material had been held under strict control by the Research Institute and not distributed elsewhere on a sufficient scale to be generally available.

Patent possibilities were not considered until the inventor (the person who actually made the attenuation discovery) had written this work up with two co-authors for publication in *Proceedings of the Society for Experimental Biology and Medicine*. The patent view taken was that the Helsinki disclosure was non-enabling and that a patent application should be filed before publication of the full paper in order to obtain patent protection for the attenuated virus and for a vaccine based on it. At this stage the virus had not been isolated from the chicken cells but the cell associated virus was considered to be useful for the purposes of a vaccine. Although the attenuation process could be reproduced from a written description it was considered desirable as a precaution to deposit the attenuated virus in a culture collection. There being no British official culture collection organised to take viruses it was decided to deposit the attenuated MD virus in a virus collection held in a laboratory of the British Ministry of Agriculture. This being done the UK patent application was filed in November 1968.

Although foreign patent applications could be delayed under the Paris Convention until the following year it was decided to file a US patent application within one year of the Helsinki meeting. The proceedings of this Congress had later become published and although oral disclosures are not as damaging as printed publications it was felt that all doubt could be eliminated by filing within the US grace period.

UK Patent 1,292,803 was later granted together with the corresponding US Patent No. 3,674,861 and patents in many other foreign countries. The UK specification is reproduced in Figs. 10.5–10.13.

This case raised the question whether it would be possible to patent a virus. The attenuated virus was new as regards the scientific literature and there was no evidence that attenuation occurred in Nature. If such a virus could be the subject of a product claim the next question was whether the claim could simply state 'attenuated MD virus' or whether it would be necessary to define the attenuated virus in some more specific way. Attenuation was accompanied by the loss of antigens one of which was known as the A antigen and it seemed likely or possible that there was a relation between these two events. This connection is cautiously stated in the specification but in the product claim to the strain (Claim 19) of the British patent the strain is defined as being substantially free of the A antigen. However, in the claim to the vaccine (Claim 25) the virus is defined as 'avian cell-attenuated'.

The USA patent application

United States patent practice in 1969 was rather strict in requiring the deposition in US culture collections of any novel organisms which were essential to the working of an invention described in a US patent application. The attempt was therefore made to transfer the cell associated virus from the British Ministry of Agriculture collection to the American Type Culture Collection before the filing of the US application. Entry of the virus into the USA was refused and the patent application was therefore filed without this safeguard. It was clear from further enquiries made later that under the health controls assiduously carried out in the USA no permit for the entry of such a virus would have been allowed, irrespective of its non-pathogenic nature. However this proved not to be serious because the inventor's specification was entirely sufficient as an enabling disclosure and the lack of a deposit was not put in issue by the US Patent Examiner.

PATENT SPECIFICATION   (11) **1 292 803**

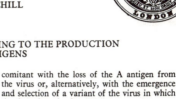

NO DRAWINGS

1292 803

(21) Application No. 54717/68   (22) Filed 18 Nov. 1968

(23) Complete Specification filed 29 Oct. 1969

(45) Complete Specification published 11 Oct. 1972

(51) International Classification A61K 23/00

(52) Index at acceptance A5B   768 76Y

(72) Inventor ANTHONY EDWARD CHURCHILL

(54) IMPROVEMENTS RELATING TO THE PRODUCTION OF ANTIGENS

(71)   We, NATIONAL RESEARCH DEVELOPMENT CORPORATION, a British Corporation established by Statute, of Kingsgate House, 66—74 Victoria Street,
5 London, S.W.1., do hereby declare the invention for which we pray that a patent may be granted to us, and the method by which it is to be performed, to be particularly described in and by the following statement: —
10   This invention relates to the production of antigenic materials and is particularly concerned with antigenic material useful in the preparation of vaccine intermediates and vaccines for the treatment or prevention of
15 Marek's disease.

Marek's disease is a disease affecting poultry and constitutes one of the most serious infectious conditions of the chicken at the present time, affecting all classes of poultry stock
20 including breeding and commercial egg producing stock and broilers. It is an infectious lymphoproliferative disease in which lymphoid tumours of the viscera are common and evidence is now available indicating that the cause
25 of the disease is a virus or virus-like agent of the herpes group. Isolation of the virus in the cell-bound state has been achieved by the present inventor and his colleagues in tissue culture experiments in which chicken kidney
30 cell monolayers are inoculated with kidney cells from diseased birds and incubated at 38.5° C. in a humified atmosphere of 5% carbon dioxide in air. From 7—10 days later, a virus-like cytopathic effect is observed, the
35 cells showing intranuclear herpes-like particles which are strongly bound within the cells and not readily separable in an infective form. (See Nature *215* 1967, 528—530).

It has now been discovered that during the
40 passage of the virus in cell culture, certain characteristics of the virus are altered. Among the most important of the changes observed is a dramatic reduction in the pathogenicity of the virus after a certain number of passages.
45 This loss of pathogenicity is thought to be con-

comitant with the loss of the A antigen from the virus or, alternatively, with the emergence and selection of a variant of the virus in which the A antigen is absent.

It has also been discovered that a A antigen- 50 depleted virus that emerges during passage still possesses other antigenic components, and furthermore, that the retained antigens give rise to antibodies which confer on birds a very significant measure of protection against chal- 55 lenge with virulent virus either by inoculation of the infective agent or by transfer thereof from bird to bird as in the course of natural infection. These observations, of the development of an immunogenic form of an oncogenic 60 virus i.e. a tumor causing virus, are quite unprecedented and lead to the possibility of producing, for the first time, a vaccine effective against such a virus.

In accordance with this invention, antigenic 65 material is obtained by passaging a pathogenic Marek's disease virus in avian cells and continuing passaging until the virus has acquired a degree of non-pathogenicity suitable for the preparation of a live vaccine. 70

The attenuated form of the virus produced by passaging in accordance with the invention also possesses other desirable characteristics in addition to its protective properties. For example, the attenuated virus has proved to be 75 remarkably stable in that it does not revert to the pathogenic state after inoculation into fowls. In addition, it provides protection not onyl against challenge with the pathogenic strain from which it was obtained but also 80 against other strains of the virus, including especially acute strains. Moreover the attenuated virus shows little tendency to spread from inoculated birds into uninoculated birds in the same flock and this is an especially important 85 advantage in the practical use of vaccines based on the live attenuated virus.

Another advantage of vaccines based on the attenuated virus is that they substantially reduce the incidence of other diseases of fowls, 90

[*Price 25p*]

particularly coccidiosis. It is thought that this reduction is due to the general improvement in health brought about by the reduction in the incidence of Marek's disease.

5   The process of this invention may be applied to any strain of Marek's disease. Especially good results are obtained with the HPRS 16 strain of the virus and since this particular strain has been extensively investigated in pre-

10 vious reasearch its use for the purpose of this invention is particularly recommended. However, various other strains of the virus are also encountered in the field and may be readily obtained from infected birds for the purposes

15 of this invention. These other strains are of varying degrees of pathogenicity but as regards cultural characteristics and all other important properties are essentially of the same type as will appear from experiments described here-

20 inafter. Thus two strains of virus, termed Frant strains, isolated from a flock of birds maintained free of certain specific pathogens, differ markedly in pathogenicity but are nevertheless capable of attenuation to produce a protective

25 form of the virus. Other strains related to HPRS 16 are, for example, the HPRS 24 and HPRS B14 strains. Similarly, strains which are available in the United States of America known as the JM, GA, CAL—1, and

30 CONN—A are also amenable to attenuation in accordance with this invention. In particular, the JM strain grows and produces a cytopathic effect similar to that of the HPRS and Frant strains and contains the same A, B

35 and C antigens. As previously stated, the virus is difficult to isolate in quantity from cells without some loss of activity and it is therefore preferred to employ cell-associated virus as the inoculum as the means for trans-

40 ferring the virus from one passage to the next.
    Many species of avian cell may be used to carry out the attenuation process including, for example, chicken, duck, quail, pheasant and turkey cells, chicken cells, being highly pre-

45 ferred. Where cell and tissue culture methods are employed, kidney cells or embryo fibroblasts have been found to be eminently successful as the host cells. For example, pathogenic virus isolated from tumours or other chicken

50 tissues may be repeatedly passaged in cultures of chicken kidney cells until the required attenuation is obtained. This usually commences between the 20th and 30th passage and it is frequently found that after, for example,

55 the 31st or the 39th passage the virus has acquired the appropriate properties for the production of a live attenuated vaccine. To ensure that a vaccine of the highest standard is obtained, the cells used for passaging are pre-

60 ferably initially free of the virus. Very encouraging results have been obtained where attenuation is in part achieved by passaging in one type of cell and completed by subsequent passes in a different type of avian cell.

65 For example, the use of chick embryo fibro-

blasts has been found to be particularly advantageous and a preferred method of performing the attenuation process comprises passaging the virus first in chick kidney or other

70 avian kidney cells followed by passaging in chick embryo fibroblasts. One of the most attractive procedures so far developed employs chick embryo fibroblasts for the majority of passages in the attenuation process. Thus the

75 pathogenic virus may undergo from about 1 to about 6 passes, preferably 3 or 4 passes, in chick kidney cells in order to adapt the virus to the cell system followed by from about 15 to about 20 passes in the chick

80 embryo fibroblasts. The employment of two types of cell system enables greater control to be exercised on the purity of the final product and the highly selective properties of the chick embryo fibroblasts for

85 Marek's disease virus are particularly important in this connection. Also, chick fibroblasts are a particularly convenient type of cell to employ on a large scale.
    The number of passages required to achieve

90 the appropriate degree of attenuation may in general be determined readily by experiment. Thus the cultures may be tested at each stage for the concomitant presence of the A antigen by means of the well known gel diffusion test

95 (Chubb and Churchill Vet. Rec. 1963, *83*, 4). It will be appreciated that the number of passages depends to some extent on the degree of pathogenicity of the original strain selected. Usually it is unnecessary to exceed about 30

100 or in some cases about 40 passages and it is frequently possible to employ a number of passages significantly lower than this especially in the preferred two stage method referred to above.

105 Cultivation of the virus in avian cells may be achieved employing a wide variety of nutrient media and very satisfactory results have been obtained with a number of standard media and modifications of these. For example,

110 Earle's balanced salt/lactalbumen hydrolysate (Medium No. 1, see Example 1) has been used with advantage. Good results have also been obtained, particularly with chick embryo fibroblast primary cultures, with the use of

115 Medium No. 2 consisting of SM 199 (84%), tryptose phosphate broth (30 g/l, 5%), calf serum (5%) and penicillin/streptomycin (as in Medium No. 1). The composition of SM 199 is given by Morgan et al, Proc. Soc. Exp. Boal.

120 Med. *73*, 1 (1950). A modification (Medium No. 3) of Medium No. 2 in which SM 199 is replaced by Eagle's medium of enhanced vitamin and aminoacid content (Macpherson et al, Virology *16*, 147 (1962)) may also be used. A

125 further modification (Medium No. 4) of Medium No. 2 is possible in which Hank's salts are used in replacement of Earle's salts.
    It will be appreciated that the process of this invention leads to the production of anti-

130 genic material in the form of an antigenic but

Fig. 10.6. Reproduced by kind permission of the Controller, H.M. Stationery Office.

1,292,803   3

non-pathogenic form of Marek's disease virus, and, concomitantly, to a protective A antigen-free strain of the virus. More particularly the antigenic material comprises avian cells containing cell-associated attenuated virus. Such material is useful as a seed material in the production of a vaccine and is embraced *per se* within the scope of the present invention. One particular class of such material comprises chicken cells containing an attenuated form of the HPRS 16 strain of the virus, and a culture of chicken kidney cells containing attenuated virus has been deposited with the collection of veterinary viruses held by the Central Veterinary Laboratory, Weybridge, Surrey, where it is identified by the code number LEU/16/AT.

In order to produce a vaccine the attenuated virus obtained as described above may be further cultivated in the same cell system as used for the attenuation process or in related systems. Thus, if desired, the virus may be transferred from one cell system to another in a later stage of the process. For example, the attenuation and multiplication of the virus may be carried out in cultured cells and the virus may then be transferred to the bloodstream of intact birds and a vaccine obtained by recovering the blood of the animals. Chick embryo liver and lung cells may also be used.

Live vaccine, containing Marek's disease virus which has become attenuated by passage in avian cells, may be administered in various ways, e.g. by subcutaneous or intramuscular injection into the young chick or into the embryo. Intramuscular injection into the leg is a particularly preferred route of administration.

The invention is illustrated in the following Examples.

Example 1

Preparation of Cell Culture:
The kidneys were dissected from one to eight week old chicks immediately after death, and finely chopped with scissors and washed three times by agitation in 20 ml. phosphate buffered saline (PBS) (pH 7.2), followed by decantation. The cells were dispersed by trypsinisation, 20 ml. of 0.05% trypsin ("Difco" Trade Mark 1:250 trypsin) in PBS being added to the chopped kidney in a conical flask. Four, five minute, cycles of trypsinisation were allowed, using fresh trypsin for each cycle and a magnetic stirrer. The cell suspension obtained from each trypsinising cycle was added to 1.0 ml. of calf serum to inhibit the trypsin, and then subjected to 5 minutes centrifugation at 1,000 r.p.m. on an MSE Minor centrifuge. The cell pellett was resuspended in cell culture growth medium (Medium No. 1) and the cells counted, using a haemocytometer. This cell suspension was diluted to contain 2 x 10⁶ cells per 5.0 ml. in growth medium.

Medium No. 1

Earle's balanced salt solution	84%	
Tryptose phosphate broth	5%	65
(30 g/litre)		
Lactalbumen hydrolysate		
(50 g/litre)	5%	
Calf serum (heat-inactivated)	5%	
Penicillin (20,000 Us/ml.)		70
)	1%	
Streptomycin (20 mg/ml.)		

2 x 10⁶ Cells in 5.0 ml. growth medium were added to each culture vessel ("Falcon" Trade Mark plastic petri-dishes—50 mm.). Cell cultures were incubated at 37—38.5° C. in a humidified atmosphere of 5% CO₂. When the monolayers were confluent, usually after 3 days incubation, the medium was charged for maintenance medium. The composition of this was the same as that given for growth medium except that the tryptose phosphate broth and the calf serum were each reduced to 2% of the total volume. Monolayers were infected on the day that they became confluent after the maintenance medium had been added.

Virus Isolation from Infected Chickens:
For this purpose the 25th chick passage of the HPRS—16 strain of Acute Marek's disease has been found satisfactory.

Ovarian lymphoid tumours were forced through a 2-inch square sterile stainless-steel gauze (gauge 978) over a petri-dish by manual pressure using a sterile spatula. The tissue passing through was suspended in PBS by being vigorously pipetted. After standing on the bench for 2 minutes in a glass container to allow the larger pieces of tissue to sediment, the supernatant cell suspension was separated and centrifuged at 1,000 r.p.m. for 10 minutes in an MSE Minor centrifuge. The cell deposit was then resuspended in a convenient volume of cell culture growth medium. The resulting suspension was next passed through a 150 gauge stainless-steel gauze in a microfilter syringe. The filtrate should consist mainly of single tumour cells. These cells were mounted in a haemocytometer and the cell concentration adjusted to about 10 x 10⁶ cells per 1.0 ml. 0.5 ml. of this cell suspension was then inoculated on to each 3 day old confluent chicken kidney monolayer. In this primary isolation passage, the cultures were incubated for a further 10 to 14 days with medium changes at 3 day intervals.

Virus Passage:
When the cytopathic effect of the virus was well developed in the cells they were removed from the surface on which they were growing by dispersion with 0.05% trypsin in "Versene" (Trade Mark) (EDTA). The suspended

Fig. 10.7 Reproduced by kind permission of the Controller, H.M. Stationery Office.

cells were spun out of the trypsin-versene mixture, resuspended in medium and used to infect fresh confluent monolayers. Owing to the fact that the virus was cell-associated, the increase in sytopathic effect from passage to passage was slow. Therefore, in the early passages the number of vessels used may be no more than doubled at each passage, but at later passages this may be improved to a four times or eight times increase in the number of cultures.

Characteristics of Attenuated Virus:
Virus continuously passaged in chicken kidney cell culture became attenuated after five to six months. Attenuated virus produced an increased rate of development of cytopathic effect such that the period between each passage was reduced from 7 days to 3 days. The attenuated virus produced macroscopic plaques 1.0—1.5 mm across, in chicken kidney monolayers in 6 to 7 days. In heavily infected cultures there was no antigen detectable by the Octerlony technique released into the culture medium, whereas in the case of non-attenuated virus, such an antigen was released. It was necessary to concentrate the medium from infected cultures up to 50 times by extraction of water or by precipitation of the antigens with ammonium sulphate to demonstrate the absence of this antigen satisfactorily.
The attenuated virus did not induce clinical Marek's disease when administered to one day old chicks of a susceptible strain (e.g. HPRS—RIR strain) by the intravenous or intra-abdominal route in the form of an infected chicken kidney cell suspension.

Production of Experimental Vaccine:
Seed virus in the form of frozen infected chicken kidney cells stored in 7.5% Dimethyl sulphoxide (DMSO) in a liquid nitrogen refrigerator was rapidly thawed and used to inoculate confluent chicken kidney monolayers. A dose of about 10^3 plaque forming units was satisfactory for each 50 mm petri-dish. These cultures were then passaged at suitable intervals (e.g. 3—6 days) according to the efficiency with which the cytopathic effect developed. The cells from each infected culture were used to infect 2 to 8 fresh cultures according to the level of cytopathic effect. After 6—10 such passages, determined according to the quantity of vaccine required, the harvested infected chicken kidney cell suspension was dispensed into ampoules and stored in 7.5% DMSO in a liquid nitrogen refrigerator. An estimate of the content of infected cells in each container was made by a plaque assay on chicken kidney monolayers.

Dose:
A suitable dilution of the stored vaccine was computed such that each chick to be vaccinated received a dose of from about 5×10^2 to about 7×10^3 plaque forming units. A suitable diluent was physiological saline buffered at pH 7.2.

Route of Administration:
Inoculation was carried out immediately after dilution of the vaccine. The vaccine was given by the intra-abdominal (intra-peritoneal) route in a volume from 0.2 to 1.0 ml, e.g. 0.5 ml. per chick.

Large Scale Production:
The virus was grown in quantity using chicken kidney monolayers grown in Roux flasks or Thompson bottles. To produce monolayer cultures in these vessels, Roux flasks were seeded with 40×10^6 freshly trypsinised chicken kidney cells in 100 ml. growth medium and Thompson bottles with 80×10^6 cells in 200 ml. In this case, the same growth and maintenance media given previously were used except that Earle's Balanced Salt Solution was replaced by Hank's Balanced Salt Solution. Virus was passaged through a sufficient number of passages usually not exceeding 10, and harvested when a sufficient number of cultures for the vaccine batch required showed cytopathic effects involving more than 10% of the cell sheet.

Storage of Vaccine:
Harvested infected cells were removed from the trypsin and versene mixture by centrifugation as previously described. The cells were then resuspended in growth medium containing 10% calf serum and 7.5% Dimethyl sulphoxide. The cell concentration was adjusted to about 4×10^6 cells per 1.0 ml., and the cell suspension dispensed into ampoules which were then sealed. The cooling rate from $+4°$ C. to $-40°$ C. was controlled at a rate of $1°$ C. per minute. After $-40°$ C. the ampoules were transferred rapidly to the liquid nitrogen refrigerator.

Tests for Immunogenicity in Chickens:
It has been found that 500—7,000 plaque forming units inoculated into chicks at one day or two weeks old produces no untoward effect in a 20 week observation period. Subsequent challenge by contract with virulent virus 3 to 4 weeks after vaccination has demonstrated solid protection in those vaccinated as against 50% or higher mortality in the unvaccinated challenged controls.
In order to provide a routine test of the immunogenicity of vaccine batches, 20 one-day old chicks should be inoculated intra-abdominally with vaccine while another 20 are held in separate isolation accommodation as unvaccinated controls. Four weeks later, both vaccinated and control chicks are challenged by inoculation with cells containing virulent virus.

Fig. 10.8. Reproduced by kind permission of the Controller, H.M. Stationery Office.

Test for Spreading:

A group of vaccinated HPRS RIR birds were left in direct contact with a group of susceptible birds and in indirect contact with a second group of susceptible birds of the same strain for 18 weeks. All groups were bled at 9 weeks, 11 weeks and 18 weeks and sera tested for antibody. At 18 weeks after vaccination all birds were bled and the buffy coats of their blood were tested for the presence of vaccine virus. The following table shows the results obtained: —

Tests for Spreading	Vaccinated	Direct Contact	Indirect Contact
Number of Birds	15	8	14
Antibody % at 11 and 18 weeks	7	0	0
Virus isolated	4	0	0

Test for Stability:

The attenuated HPRS 16 strain was tested for stability by isolating the virus from the blood of 7 viraemic chickens, 15 weeks after inoculation at one day of age with HPRS 16, 39th passage. The buffy coat from these 8 blood samples was cooled and inoculated into 15 one day old HPRS—RIR chickens. During an 18 weeks observation period these birds remained clinically normal. Virus isolated from the circulation of two of these chicks showed the characteristic absence of the A antigen of attenuated virus.

Example 2

Isolation and attenuation:

A strain of Marek's disease virus of low natural pathogenicity was isolated from kidneys of 4 week old chickens of a 'Specific Pathogen Free' breeding flock maintained in isolation and freedom from antibody to leucocis, avian encephalomyelitis, infectious bronchitis, Newcastle disease, infectious laryngotracheitis, CELO and GAL viruses, *Mycoplasma gallisepticum* and *S. pullorum*.

The kidneys were trypsinised and grown in the Earle's-lactalbumen medium, as described in Example 1. Cytopathic effect, typical of Marek's disease microplaques, was observed microscopically. The virus was then passaged 12 times in chicken kidney cell cultures on Medium No. 3, 12 times in chicken embryo fibroblast on Medium No. 3, and further 12 times in duck embryo fibroblast cultures on Medium No. 3. The virus strain so obtained was tested by gel diffusion and was shown to have lost its "A" antigen.

Tests for pathogenicity:

a) 50 (one day old) 'Sykes Line 50' genetically susceptible chickens, possessing maternal antibody, were inoculated with $10^{4.5}$ plaque forming units (pfu) of the attenuated Frant Strain per bird intra-muscularly. These animals showed no clinical symptoms for eleven months. They laid fertile eggs, of which over 100 were hatched and the chickens kept and observed for signs of the disease. Histological specimens of seven birds of the inoculated group were shown to be free of the lesions of Marek's disease.

b) Similar experiments using 20 'Sykes Line 50' chickens (day old), having maternal antibody, were carried out by inoculating the birds with 10^3 pfu doses and similar results were obtained.

c) A group of genetically susceptible HPRS 'Rhode Island Red Chickens', having maternal antibody, were inoculated with 10^4 pfu doses per bird. These birds were found to be clinically normal 12 weeks after inoculation.

d) Four groups of 10 Brown Leghorn chickens, free of antibody, were inoculated with approximately 10^4 pfu dosages per bird. They remained clinically normal for six weeks, were sacrificed, and showed no macroscopic lesions.

Tests for immunogenicity:

a) A group of day-old 'Sykes Line 50' chickens was inoculated as follows: 27 with 10^4 pfu of the 36th passage of the virus per bird, 10 days later, the inoculated group together with two control groups of 27 and 25 birds, respectively, were challenged by inoculation with a dosage of 150 pfu of the 7th passage level of the HPRS 16 virus strain per bird. The mortalities observed six months later were as follows:

Fig. 10.9. Reproduced by kind permission of the Controller, H.M. Stationery Office.

Group	Inoculated	Control	Control
Number of birds	27	27	25
Number of birds died	5	27	21

The results show that the inoculated group was protected and a high percentage of the birds survived the inoculated challenge.

5   b) In a further experiment groups of 20 'Sykes Line 50' chickens (day-old) were inoculated with different doses of the attenuated Frant and HPRS 16 viruses. After 20 days the birds together with unvaccinated controls, were challenged intra-muscularly with 10 the unattenuated strain of HPRS 16 by using dosage of 10^2 pfu per bird. All birds were killed after 5 months and subjected to macroscopic examination for lesions.

The results were as follows: 15

Dose pfu/bird	Frant attenuated strain			HPRS 16 attenuated strain		Controls	
	9×10^3	9×10^2	9×10	3×10^2	3×10		
Number of birds	20	20	20	20	20	20	10
Number of birds with lesions	2	5	15	5	12	20	8

c) In order to find the best possible dosage necessary to protect the birds against natural forms of infection, groups of 20 of the same
20 type of chickens were inoculated with the attenuated Frant Strain at various dosage levels, and challenged by keeping them in contact with a group of other 20 birds previously inoculated with 100 pfu per bird of the unattenuated acute HPRS 16 strain, to provide 25 a source of infection. All birds were killed after five months, and the following tabulated results show the incidence of Marek's disease in the relevant groups:

Dose pfu/bird	10^3	10^2	10	None Control	Source Birds
Number of birds	20	20	20	20	20
Number of birds with lesions	0	2	8	17	20

It is clear that a dosage of 1,000 pfu per bird provided adequate protection against infection from other birds in the flock.

with the isolated strain remained clinically normal for at least 6 months, which indicated that there was no reversal to the pathogenic form. 45

Test for stability
35 The attenuated Frant Strain was tested for stability by isolating the virus from the blood of one 'Sykes Line 50' chicken inoculated in the tests for absence of pathogenicity, and growing the virus on a Marek's disease free
40 chicken kidney culture. Tissue culture tests showed that the strain had no "A" antigen. 20 'Sykes Line 50' day-old chickens inoculated

Test for oncogenicity:
Hamster cheek pouch tests were carried out according to the recognised method. None of the animals receiving the attenuated strain in association with chicken embryo fibroblast 50 cells showed any symptoms. These results were confirmed in two groups of three newborn hamsters, which showed no clinical symptoms after 8 weeks of treatment.

Fig. 10.10. Reproduced by kind permission of the Controller, H.M. Stationery Office.

Tests for spreading

A group of vaccinated 'Sykes Line 50' birds were left in contact with susceptible birds for 4 months. Both groups were bled fortnightly
5 and their sera tested for antibody and for presence of vaccine virus. At 11 weeks after vaccination all birds were bled and buffy coats of their blood were tested for presence of vaccine virus. The following table shows the results obtained:
10

	Vaccinated with 10⁵ pfu/bird	In-contacts
Number of birds	5	10
Antibody detected	*All* positive at 10 weeks	*None* positive at 4 months
Virus isolated	3	0

Test for protection against different acute virus:

15 3 Groups of 18 Brown Leghorn Marek's disease free birds were selected. The first group was inoculated with an acute unattenuated 'Frant No. 2' strain isolated under circumstances independent and unrelated to the
20 isolation of the Frant strain hereinbefore described. Each bird received 500 pfu of the 'Frant No. 2' virus, and was used as a contact challenge for susceptible controls (Group 2) and a third group vaccinated with 1,000 pfu per bird of the attenuated Frant strain.
25 The birds were bled at intervals and their sera tested for antibodies to the vaccine and to the challenged 'Frant No. 2' viruses. Eight weeks after the experiment had commenced only two of the vaccinated birds had antibody to the
30 challenged viruses, whereas eight of eleven control birds had such antibody. The experiment had also shown that unattenuated strains would spread freely to any contacts, as expected from experience in the field.

35 *Tests for suitability for use as a vaccine:*

Passages of the Frant strain were tested for mycoplasma and were found to be free of such contamination. Field trials were then carried out with a vaccine containing the Frant
40 attenuated strain in a cell-associated form with chicken embryo fibroblast cells, involving several thousand birds. The vaccine (0.2ml, 10³ pfu) was injected intramuscularly into the leg of the bird. In each case half of the flock
45 was inoculated with 1,000 pfu intramuscularly. Whenever there was incidence of Marek's disease in uninoculated birds in the flock, those having received the vaccine remained unaffected.

50 **Example 3**

Experiment with the HPRS 16 Strain:

This strain, after 15 passages according to Example 1, was further passaged 12 times in chicken kidney cells, on Medium No. 1, 12

times in chicken embryo fibroblast cells on
55 Medium No. 3, and 12 times in duck embryo fibroblast cells on Medium No. 3. The strain was then tested in 10 'Sykes Line 50' day-old chickens, which were inoculated with 10³ pfu of the strain and later observed clinically for
60 six months. No symptoms appeared and there was a complete absence of lesions when subjecting all birds to a postmortem examination.

Example 4

Experiments with the 'Frant No. 2' Strain:
65 This highly pathogenic strain, called the 'Frant No. 2' strain, was first adapted to chicken kidney cells by three passages in such cultures on Medium No. 3, and was attenuated by a further 15 passages in chicken em-
70 bryo fibroblast primary cultures using Media Nos. 2 and 3. The strain was shown to have completely lost its "A"antigen, and was apathogenic, immunogenic and safe for use in vaccines according to tests already described.
75

Example 5

The JM strain of Marek's disease virus is attenuated by passage in chick kidney cells (3 passes using Medium No. 1) followed by passage in duck embryo fibroblast (3 passes)
80 using Medium No. 3. Finally the strain is given from 15 to 18 passes in chick embryo fibroblast using Medium No. 2. The attenuated strain so obtained is free of the A antigen and is of very high purity. Leucosis
85 agents and other contaminant materials sometimes present in the chick kidneys are removed by selection in the subsequent passes in duck and chick fibroblast cells. The strain is tested according to the procedures given in
90 Example 2 and shown to be highly satisfactory for the purposes of a vaccine.

Example 6

The procedure described in Example 5 is followed using strains GA, CAL—1, and
95 CONN—A separately to produce attenuated

Fig. 10.11. Reproduced by kind permission of the Controller, H.M. Stationery Office.

virus. Each attenuated virus is processed into vaccine form.

Example 7

5 This Example describes the results of several large scale trials made using the vaccine prepared as described in Example 1.

Day-old and three week old chicks were vaccinated by the intra-abdominal (intra-peritoneal) route with a single dose of the vaccine prepared from attenuated strain of HPRS 16. 10 Each chick was given a dose of from 0.2 to 1.0 mol. of the vaccine. The chicks were kept under normal field conditions for a period of 235 days. The incidence of Marek's disease and other non-specified diseases, particularly 15 coccidiosis, in the vaccinated chicks and in unvaccinated control groups are given in the following tables:—

1st Trial:

	Day old		3 weeks old		Unvaccinated	
Total number	1,000		1,000		2,000	
Total mortality	5	0.05%	8	0.08%	42	2.1%
Marek's disease mortality	0	0%	0	0%	17	0.85%
Non-specified disease mortality	5	0.05%	8	0.08%	25	1.25%

2nd Trial:

	Day old		3 weeks old		Unvaccinated	
Total number	1,250		1,250		2,500	
Total mortality	18	1.44%	19	1.52%	67	2.68%
Marek's disease mortality	1	0.08%	1	0.08%	7	0.28%
Non-specified disease mortality	17	1.36%	18	1.44%	60	2.4%

3rd Trial: 3 weeks old

	Vaccinated		Unvaccinated	
Total number	879		2,700	
Total mortality	29	3.24%	443	16.4%
Marek's disease mortality	9	1.03%	115	4.3%
Non-specified disease mortality	20	2.21%	328	12.1%

4th Trial: 3 weeks old

	Vaccinated		Unvaccinated	
Total number	900		6,100	
Total mortality	36	4%	1,789	29.3%
Marek's disease mortality	12	1.33%	1,076	17.6%
Non-specified disease mortality	24	2.67%	713	11.7%

Fig. 10.12. Reproduced by kind permission of the Controller, H.M. Stationery Office.

WHAT WE CLAIM IS:—

1. Process for the production of antigenic material which comprises passaging Marek's disease virus in avian cells until the virus is sufficiently attenuated for use in a live vaccine.

2. Process according to Claim 1, in which passaging is continued until the virus is substantially free of the A antigen.

3. Process according to Claim 1 or 2, in which the avian cells used are chicken cells or duck cells.

4. Process according to Claim 3 in which the cells are kidney cells.

5. Process according to Claim 3, in which the cells are fibroblasts.

6. Process according to any of Claims 1 to 5, in which the virus is passaged in one species of avian cell and then in another species of avian cell.

7. Process according to Claim 6, in which the virus is first passaged in chick embryo kidney cells and subsequently passaged in chick embryo fibroblast and/or duck embryo fibroblasts.

8. Process according to Claim 7, in which the number of passages in the fibroblasts exceeds that in the kidney cells.

9. Process according to any of the preceding Claims, in which the total number of passages is at least 20.

10. Process according to Claim 9, in which the number of passages is at least 25.

11. Process according to Claim 10, in which the number of passages is from 31 to 39.

12. Process according to Claim 8, in which the number of passages in kidney cells is from 1 to 6.

13. A process in which Marek's disease virus attenuated according to any of the preceding Claims is formulated into a vaccine for parenteral administration.

14. Process for the production of a vaccine active against Marek's disease which comprises inoculating avian cells with an avian cell-associated pathogenic form of Marek's disease virus, passaging the virus in one or more species of avian cell until it has lost the A antigen and thereafter formulating the attenuated virus into a vaccine for parenteral administration.

15. Process according to Claim 14, in which the total number of passages between the original strain and the vaccine strain of virus is at least 20.

16. Process according to any of the preceding Claims, in which the strain of virus subjected to passaging is the HPRS 16 strain.

17. Process according to any of Claims 1 to 15, in which the strain of virus subjected to passaging is a Frant strain.

18. Process according to any of Claims 1 to 15, in which the strain of virus subjected to passaging is selected from the JM, GA, CAL—1 and CONN—A strains.

19. A strain of Marek's disease virus substantially free of the A antigen.

20. Avian cells containing a cell-associated antigenic but non-pathogenic form of Marek's disease virus.

21. Cells according to Claim 20, being chick kidney cells.

22. Cells according to Claim 20, being chick embryo fibroblasts.

23. Cells according to Claim 20 in association with water or other physiologically acceptable diluent.

24. Chicken kidney cells containing attenuated Marek's disease virus having the characteristics of the cells indentified by No. LEU/16/AT held by the Central Veterinary Laboratory, Weybridge, Surrey, England.

25. A live vaccine protective against Marek's disease comprising as an antigenic component an avian cell-attenuated form of Marek's disease virus.

26. A vaccine according to Claim 25, containing from about 5 x 10² to about 7 x 10³ plaque forming units per unit dose.

27. A method of protecting poultry against Marek's disease which comprises inoculating the chick embryo or the young chick with a live vaccine as defined in Claim 25 or 26.

28. A method according to Claim 27, in which the vaccine is given by subcutaneous or intramuscular injection.

29. A method according to Claim 27, in which the vaccine is injected into the leg of the chick.

30. A method according to Claim 27, in which the vaccine is given by intra-abdominal injection.

31. A method according to Claim 27, in which the poultry are susceptible to Marek's disease and coccidiosis and are thereby protected against both infections.

R. S. CRESPI.
Chartered Patent Agent
Agent for the Applicants.

Printed for Her Majesty's Stationery Office by the Courier Press, Leamington Spa, 1972. Published by the Patent Office, 25 Southampton Buildings, London, WC2A 1AY, from which copies may be obtained.

Fig. 10.13. Reproduced by kind permission of the Controller, H.M. Stationery Office.

The first US application having been filed as a precaution it was decided some months later to file a second patent application as a continuation-in-part of the first. This enabled additional experimental data to be included to update the specification with the best possible disclosure. The second application was filed within one year of the British priority date and was thereby enabled to take advantage for priority purposes of both the British application and the first US application. Later the first US application was allowed to lapse in favour of the continuation-in-part application.

The US patent was granted without extraordinary difficulty. However the Examiner would not allow any claim to a virus. At this date there was considerable doubt in US professional circles whether claims to micro-organisms and viruses would be legally valid and since the Examiner appeared to be favourable to the other claims it was decided not to contest this issue. The US Examiner required a much more detailed attenuation process claim than had been found acceptable elsewhere. Usually the more detailed a claim the narrower is its scope but in this case the extra detail was explanatory rather than restrictive and so it was decided to accord with the Examiner's wishes. The Examiner allowed a product-by-process claim to a vaccine based on the attenuated virus substantially free of the A antigen when produced by the process covered in the main attenuation process claim.

Shortly before the US claims were finalised it was discovered that US research workers had developed a competitive vaccine based on a strain of virus isolated from turkeys and not from chickens. This was known as turkey herpes virus (HTV). A vaccine based on the HTV virus was later patented as UK 1,316,168 and corresponding US Patent 3,642,574 with equivalents in other countries. The patents stress the fact that HTV virus was non-pathogenic in Nature, did not require attenuation and had not lost its A antigen. The US patent states that the HTV virus can be released from cells, e.g. by sonication, and that this differentiates it from MD virus. Curiously, this disclosure is absent from the corresponding British patent.

It was now prudent to consider the possible relationship between the two developments. Could the claims of the MD vaccine patent application be amended, even at this late stage, so as to be relevant to the competitive vaccine? By this time more scientific knowledge was available on the importance or otherwise of the A antigen. In retrospect, it was considered that it would have been better to describe the loss of the A antigen from the MD virus as coincidental rather than concomitant with the loss of pathogenicity. It was now concluded that the MD vaccine claims had been so strongly wedded to the loss of the A antigen that it would be a practical impossibility to move away from this restriction upon which the US Examiner had insisted. Furthermore it was fair to regard the HTV research as based on an original discovery totally independent of the work on MD virus. Therefore no change was proposed. It should be noted that a certain amount of re-wording of claims while the application is in a malleable state is perfectly legitimate. It is virtually certain that the US Examiner saw the presence or absence of the A antigen as a distinguishing feature which would allow him to grant both the patent on the MD vaccine and the patent on the HTV vaccine.

The British patent application

Examination of the patent application by the British Patent Office was straightforward. However, when the application was accepted and published it was immediately opposed by a Japanese University Research Association. At this date the practice under British law was to publish an accepted application and allow three months for interested parties to enter formal opposition to the grant of a patent on any of the specific grounds provided by law. This has now changed and under modern practice the patent is granted and a period of nine months is available for third parties to apply to have it revoked.

The Opponents cited the original *Nature* paper describing the identification of the MD virus and other publications in the scientific literature also reporting on the isolation and identification of the viral agent. These publications described the propagation of the virus in cell culture but gave no indication of attenuation or of any other fundamental change in properties. No doubt realising that these publications alone would not amount to a sufficiently strong attack against the application the Opponents also cited the full paper by the inventor and his colleagues describing the attenuation of the virus. The patent application had been filed before this paper was published but the Opponents argued that the paper submitted had been accepted by the journal prior to the applicant's filing date and that therefore it must be considered as effectively published as of the date of acceptance of the paper by the editor. To rebut this argument evidence was produced in the form of a declaration by the editor of the journal concerning confidentiality and the nature of the conditions under which prospective authors, editors and the referees operate during the period between the submission of a paper and its ultimate issuance in printed form. The evidence established that even after acceptance of the paper the editor was not totally free to disclose the information otherwise than through a channel of publication confined to the journal. No contrary evidence was brought forward and it was concluded that publication of the inventor's paper had not occurred until its actual distribution in print (the June 1969 issue of the *Journal of General Virology*). Even if the decision had been otherwise on this point the applicant would have been saved by appealing to the grace period provision which existed in British patent law at that date whereby publications in the transactions of Learned Societies would be discounted provided a patent application was filed within six months of publication. This fall-back position was also argued successfully by the applicant.

The Opponents also challenged patentability on the grounds of obviousness by arguing that once the viral nature of the disease was established and the infectious agent isolated it would be an obvious step for the skilled worker or research team in this field to proceed to the production of an attenuated strain of virus from which to prepare a suitable vaccine. Both sides brought forward expert witnesses to deal with this point based on what was known for the attenuation of other viruses in the prior art. The applicant's evidence was more decisive on these questions. First the early publications had not actually shown isolation of the causative agent and its categorical identification as a virus. Moreover, as stated in the patent application, the MD virus was oncogenic and there was no previous example of a vaccine which would protect against the formation of tumours. Again, the MD virus remained cell-associated and there was no precedent for the development of a successful vaccine from a virus which remained cell-associated.

The British Patent Office decided that the subject matter of this application was not clearly obvious over all the prior art relied upon by the Opponents and the Opposition therefore failed. Under the then prevailing law it was the practice of the Patent Office to decide in favour of applicants, especially on the issue of obviousness, where any doubt attached to the case or any important argument was not sufficiently supported by evidence.

Case study 3: tetracycline patent litigation

This is a short account of a case decided in the United Kingdom High Court in 1973 (American Cyanamid Co. v. Berk Pharmaceuticals Ltd).

The antibiotic Aureomycin had previously been produced by a strain of *Streptomyces* designated A-377, an isolate which was given the name *Streptomyces aureofaciens*. This was the type strain. Aureomycin is chlortetracycline and by chemical removal of the chlorine atom tetracycline is formed. It was later found that tetracycline itself could also be produced by *Streptomyces aureofaciens* and it became desirable to produce tetracycline to the exclusion of chlortetracycline.

The process of the American Cyanamid Patent UK 952,820 was directed to producing tetracycline by cultivating 'a strain of *Streptomyces aureofaciens* which produces tetracycline to the substantial exclusion of chlortetracycline' and these strains were characterised later in the claim by reference to a harvest mash reflectance curve and a parameter which became known as delta R, which was defined by numerical limitations. One question was whether the strain defined meant any strain of the species or simply any descendant of A-377. The defendants argued that the claim was limited to strains which were descendants of A-377 whereas the plaintiffs argued for a broader interpretation and asserted a distinction between those passages in the specification which relate to the invention in the sense of the monopoly claimed and those which relate merely to the discovery on which the invention is based.

The court held that if the broad construction of the claim were adopted the patent must be bad on its face because it told you nothing about what you may expect from or do with any strains other than descendants of A-377. The delta R test was of value only in deciding whether a strain fell within the claim but was not a test which would be of any help to anyone searching for a suitable strain. There was no fair basis for so broad a claim as the plaintiffs contended for. The defendants had pleaded that a claim of this type was no more than a statement of a known desideratum. The Judge considered this argument together with the objection of obviousness and held that the evidence showed that everyone agreed that a high tetracycline-yielding strain was one for which it was obvious enough to look even though there could be no certainty that anybody making the attempt would succeed. The test of inventive step in the present case was:

'Would the notional research group working in the field of antibiotic production at the date of the patent in all the circumstances which include . . .

(a) a knowledge of all the relevant prior art

(b) a knowledge of the past successes achieved by mutation selection programmes

(c) a knowledge of the fact that strains of *Streptomyces* designated as *Streptomyces aureofaciens* had been shown to co-produce TC and CTC in varying proportions

(d) a knowledge of the results claimed in respect of TC production in a chloride containing fermentation medium by other research teams

(e) a knowledge of the fact that TC had medical and therapeutical advantages over CTC and of the fact that a direct fermentation production method could be expected to result in cost savings . . .

directly be led as a matter of course to try to find or induce a novel strain of *Streptomyces aureofaciens* descended from A-377 – in the expectation that a strain might be found or induced which could be used in a direct fermentation process in a chloride containing medium so as to produce a very high percentage of TC in proportion to CTC, or alternatively so as to produce TC to the exclusion or substantial exclusion of CTC?'

The judge considered that the question really boiled down to how much research would be necessary to find the desired process or article, and said that a patient searcher is as much entitled to a monopoly as someone who hits upon an invention by some lucky chance or inspiration. If the expectation of success was sufficiently predictable and the effort involved was not going to be very great then it might well be that no patentable invention could result. If the expectation was doubtful and the effort great then a person undertaking the work should be entitled to a monopoly but 'only for what he has done unless he is working in some entirely new field'. The Judge held that even if the claim was limited to descendants of A-377 it still went far beyond the patentee's entitlement because they had taught nothing more than the fact that success which had already been achieved by other workers on the same lines (i.e. to reduce the relative yield of chlortetracycline and move nearer towards the intended aim) could be extended further. The real objection to the claim was rooted in lack of fair basis because, as regards the use of strains other than the novel strains specifically disclosed, the public would be in no better position than they were before the patent was published.

The sufficiency of disclosure objection was that no information had been given to enable a skilled man to produce and identify suitable strains of *Streptomyces aureofaciens* even if the claim was limited to descendants of A-377. The delta R test was generally held to be non-viable and indeed misleading and some of the witnesses had said that they were unable to deal with delta R which they felt was of no practical importance to anyone other than those taking out patents. It appears that the delta R feature was an arbitrary one decided upon when the application was drafted and it was thought that some test for the purposes of definition was necessary. The delta R parameter seemed to be common to the strains which had been produced. This was an instructive case on the problem of claim drafting and the possible pitfalls in settling on some second order properties or parameters which are used as substitutes for the ultimate functional test itself. The broad strain definition was rejected by the court and it was held that protection was possible only for the use of the specific strains developed and deposited by the patentee.

The case is also a valuable one on the question of proving infringement by the use of strains of micro-organism which are alleged to be the same as or related to or derived from the strains disclosed in the specification. There was in this case a real conflict of evidence as to whether the defendant's strain was derived by mutation from a parent strain which both sides agreed was not *Streptomyces aureofaciens*. The defendants claimed that they made tetracycline from a mutant strain they themselves had deposited in a culture collection and which had itself been derived by a series of mutations from another deposited strain named *Streptomyces lusitanus* var. *tetracyclini*. Both sides had agreed that the latter strain was different from the *aureofaciens* strain. The plaintiff's experts, however, had carried out experiments on the defendants' mutant and claimed that it was in fact a *Streptomyces aureofaciens*. The Judge accepted the defendants' evidence as to the origin of their own strain even though this was asserted to be theoretically impossible by the plaintiff's expert witnesses. The Judge was very much influenced by the evidence of a witness who observed that it was impossible to state the derivation of any mutant unless you have direct proof of its ancestry because changes brought about by mutations may be of so radical a nature that the resulting mutant may differ so widely from the parent strain that if one were to test it from the point of view of speciation merely by the characteristics which it exhibited one might easily arrive at an entirely wrong result.

11 Biotechnology and patent protection: critique and conclusions

What conclusions can be drawn about the way the patent system works for inventions in biotechnology? This question was investigated in depth in 1985 by the Organisation for Economic Cooperation and Development (OECD). The OECD report on '*Biotechnology and Patent Protection: an international review*' was the second in a series of reports to be published by OECD on aspects of biotechnology and is one of the recommendations for further reading listed at the end of this book. This enquiry was limited to member states of the OECD but subsequently the World Intellectual Property Organisation (WIPO) extended its own enquiry world-wide and set up a 'Committee of Experts' to review the law and to meet annually for discussion. The membership of this Committee consists predominantly of Patent Office representatives from all countries which consider the subject important from their point of view. Representatives from industry and other interested circles are invited to attend as observers and are allowed to comment on the proposals and the discussions.

To answer this question further involves a critique of the existing patent system. The critique which follows is based mainly on the OECD conclusions and recommendations.

The OECD investigation extended over a wide range of complex and controversial issues. In classical biotechnology trade secrecy has often provided sufficient protection for the industrial innovator but for biotechnology in its modern phase patent protection is considered by many to make a significant contribution to scientific and business enterprise. Scientists and businessmen look to the patent law to provide forms of protection properly geared to the emerging ideas, processes, and products of this new technology. But patent law has traditions which predate the current interest in biotechnology by a considerable margin, and it must cope with the broader range of inventions which come within its sphere. The living nature of the entities involved in inventions of the microbiological type can be identified as the major single cause of tensions between the aims of applicants for patents in this field and the principles of the patent law which have in essentials remained unchanged from previous times. In applying these to biotechnology inventions, however, the diversity of opinion one encounters is truly remarkable.

The following topics deserve re-examination:

1. Whether biotechnology innovation justifies quite separate treatment and forms of patent law or can be coped with by relatively minor modifications of existing laws and regulations.

2. The absolute novelty principle in patent law which imposes constraints keenly felt by certain categories of inventor, notably those whose primary work is in academic research.

3. The patentability of micro-organisms, including the specific problem of naturally occurring as opposed to man-made organisms. Of particular concern to this question is the distinction between 'discovery' and 'invention' which is in need of clarification and international consensus.

4. (a)   The deposition of micro-organisms in culture collections and the conditions of release to third parties.

   (b)   Deposition as a possible method of solving the problem of reproducibility of the written disclosure.

5. The forms of legal protection available for new plants, especially those produced with the aid of genetic engineering techniques.

6. The time-scales of patenting procedure and the legal enforcement process.

7. The problem of education and awareness of basic patent law among research workers, especially those in the academic community, and their attitudes to the patent system.

These topics invite the following observations.

1   The adequacy of the present system

This writer believes that the structure of patent law is basically sound and generally adequate for inventions in biotechnology even though special areas of difficulty exist. There is firm official disapproval of the notion of a separate patent law for biotechnology and such a proposal is not supported by industry or other interested circles. Patent protection has an important function and cannot be dismissed in favour of commercial secrecy except in very special circumstances. Industry itself is clear as to this conclusion and, claiming control over the activities of its employee inventors, can decide to patent or to maintain secrecy case by case. The appearance on the patent scene of the academic research worker complicates the situation to some extent. Hitherto many academic research workers have either boycotted the patent system on point of principle or, having found it incompatible with their main aims, have played little part in its development leaving patents as the almost exclusive domain of industry. This state of affairs is undesirable.

Although separate legislation for biotechnology may be unnecessary it is essential that those who administer the patent system become more open to the needs of innovators in this particular technology and adapt official practices in ways which encourage use of the patent system. Patent law should offer flexibility if it is to justify its existence as supportive of advances in technology.

2   **Possible adaptation of the patent law concept of novelty**

The fundamental principle of absolute novelty in certain national laws and in the European patent law, to which the only present exceptions made include publication in evident abuse of the rights of the applicant (such as breach of confidence) and through display at officially recognised special types of international exhibition, constitutes a serious challenge to the natural desires of many research workers to achieve the earliest possible dissemination of knowledge about new discoveries of importance to science and technology. It is axiomatic that knowledge which is already in the free possession of the public cannot subsequently be withdrawn from the public domain and made the subject of any monopoly right. However this principle of preserving the rights of the public would not be seriously breached by devising a limited exception in respect of the inventor's *own* discovery which becomes known to the public *only* as a result of the contribution of the inventor himself.

The lack of any grace period in the law prevailing in Western Europe contrasts with the generous grace periods available under the patent laws of the United States of America and Canada. This is the first imbalance which might be addressed. There is already a movement towards this end under sponsorship by WIPO but industry is split on the issue. Academic workers would in general support this proposal as also would many industrial firms who have strong links with academic institutions. Also it would appeal to certain sections of the engineering industry where some degree of public use of an invention as part of reasonable trial and experiment is necessary before reaching the stage when patenting can be commenced with confidence. WIPO is sympathetic to the idea of an International Convention which would provide a grace period of at least six months (preferably 12 months) for public disclosure or use of any kind made by the inventor (alone or with co-authors or collaborators) or made by others with the inventor's evident consent and backing. It would be an essential element of this proposal that the disclosure stems directly from the inventor's work and not from independent research by third parties. It is recognised that this would introduce an exception to the current definition of the 'state of the art' deriving from the Strasbourg Convention and now embedded in European patent law as well as national laws already harmonised therewith but this alone cannot be a serious objection. Some official industrial property spokesmen have gained the impression that European industry is generally unfavourable to a grace period provision on the ground that it would cause uncertainty in the assessment of the state-of-the-art. But this objection is of dubious force and could be deflected in the grace period legislation itself. In any case the grace period available under US law appears to cause no such problems.

The likely effectiveness of grace periods having the contemplated duration is nevertheless a matter for debate in the context of biotechnology inventions. A grace period would enable an inventor to obtain a patent position after an inadvertent disclosure of an invention which is *mature* in patent terms. However it might fail to achieve its purpose where substantial further development of a published initial discovery is necessary to achieve an adequate disclosure for patent purposes. The subject is worthy of further study and should not be dismissed as something of interest only to an insignificant minority. In relation to innovation in biotechnology, inventors in academic institutions are neither insignificant nor a minority.

3   The patentability of micro-organisms

Following the precedent set in United States jurisdiction and in the practice of the European Patent office there is a clear trend towards the general acceptability of patent claims to new (man-made) micro-organisms in the form of the organism *per se*. It is desirable that this trend continue and be extended to countries which at present forbid claims to micro-organisms in *per se* or any other form.

On the patentability of naturally occurring micro-organisms the present wide spectrum of opinion is unsatisfactory. Negative attitudes appear either to be due to a questionable application of the criterion of novelty or to be based on a particularly strained interpretation of the term 'discovery' as differentiated from 'invention'. The issue is also clouded by the concept of 'product of nature' and the development of case law around this theme especially in USA. It is applied to non-living as well as to living matter although its emotive force in recent times has been experienced most in the field of micro-organism patents. It would be a welcome development if 'product of nature', as a ground of objection, could be removed from the patent law in official and judicial thought. This proposition can be defended on the basis of a 'state of the art' approach. The research worker who discovers, isolates and first makes available a new enzyme, hormone, vitamin or any other type of natural product having valuable biological properties should be allowed to obtain patent protection for it in *per se* terms. The act of first discovery, isolation and identification of a valuable naturally occurring micro-organism with a clear disclosure of industrial applicability or utility should also be recognised as an invention worthy of patent protection in the form of a *per se* claim. This should be done without resort to a limitation as to biological purity. Such limitations should be restricted to the necessary cases in which prior art disclosures exist which require the claims to be distinguished therefrom in order to meet the requirements of novelty and inventiveness over the *known* art.

4   Deposition of micro-organisms in culture collections

In United States patent practice most of the major problems of adequacy and reproducibility of disclosure and of the release of deposited micro-organisms to third parties appeared to have been solved by the Argoudelis decision. Subsequent case law has in fact been necessary to clarify certain open questions but the obligations upon the applicant are now well established. By contrast European patent law with its unhesitating adoption of the dual publication system has given rise to controversy.

(i)   *Introduction of early publication in national laws*

Mounting delays in the disclosure of patent information to the public eventually became intolerable in certain national patent circles and hence arose the practice of publishing unexamined patent applications at about 18 months after the priority date claimed under the Paris Convention. This development appeared to be a natural one and it was brought about largely without protest. From the point of view of any single industrial applicant there is presumably more to be gained from advance knowledge of the research activities of all one's competitors than is to be lost by the early disclosure of one's own research. Nevertheless the traditional 'bargain theory' of patent law had been breached in that the disclosure was now made not *in return* for the grant of protection but *in advance* of such protection and *irrespective* of whether any protection would in fact be obtained.

Early publication was an ideal early warning system. Imperceptibly, however, the alerting function of this publication became overshadowed by the idea that it should also constitute an enabling disclosure which could be utilised by the public. This again appears to have taken place without any legal justification.

(ii)   *Adoption of early publication in the European Patent Convention*

The early publication practice was taken into the European Patent Convention without question. As a corollary, Rule 28 of the Regulations provided that a deposited culture required under the Rule must also be made available to the public at the early publication date. Rule 28 was amended in June 1980 to provide a measure of control over the availability of the deposited culture in the interim between early publication of the application and grant of the European patent. In this interim the applicant has the option of specifying that release of samples must be through the intermediary of an independent expert acting for the applicant's competitor or other third party. At present applicants must contend in different countries with different types of regulation covering the release of micro-organisms deposited for patent purposes. These have been discussed in Chapter 6.

(iii)   *Variation in national practice*

Some national patent regulations have also been amended to harmonise with the current European practice, e.g. in France and Sweden, but complete unanimity among the contracting States of the European Convention has not yet emerged on this issue. The arguments for reform of national rules corresponding to the original Rule 28 provision of unrestricted availability of cultures to the public at the early publication stage have failed so far to budge certain official circles which remain anchored to the bedrock principle of the equality of all types of patent application in relation to the informational purpose of the patent system. This principle, it is alleged, makes it necessary to put microbiological inventions on the same footing as all others in regard to the effectiveness of the publication of the corresponding specification. This proposition is incontrovertible when applied to the act of final publication upon grant of the patent, but not so convincing when applied to the first or early publication of the unexamined patent application at the 18 month stage after the date of the first application in a Convention country.

(iv)   *Equality of treatment*

In order to put all applicants on the same footing as regards the informational function of the patent disclosure the microbiological applicant is obliged to meet a requirement of a kind which is imposed on no other applicant. In no other case must an applicant put into the hands of third parties from any corner of the world what is in effect an unlimited supply of the physical means of producing the benefits of the invention with relatively little effort on the part of such persons. In seeking amendment of original Rule 28 interested circles had requested a territorial limitation on the availability of these cultures. It seems hardly fair that the deposited micro-organisms should be available to all and sundry in countries having no connection whatsoever with the patent application(s) for which the deposit was necessary. This request was not accepted, however, because it was considered to be too restricted in outlook and inconsistent with the idea of openness of attitude to countries outside Europe.

The informational purpose of the patent system constitutes only one side of the coin. Moreover it is itself integrally connected with and consequential upon the other fundamental purpose of patents which is to give proper protection to the inventor. Complete equality of treatment is impossible in the very nature of the case. Informational equality can only be achieved by demanding something extra from the applicant as regards the contributive aspect of the bargain. This is true even of the later stage at which an enforceable right is granted but it applies even more so at the earliest stage of publication at which the applicant is exposed to the risk of competitive research activity which may ultimately result in a circumvention of the protection he may obtain.

There is a natural tendency for Patent Offices to attempt to restrict the applicant to protection only for the micro-organism strains deposited in a culture collection or described in the patent specification, leaving open the possibility for competitors to mutate the deposited strains and to allege that they are outside the scope of the applicant's patent. Thus in the United States an enlarged Board of Appeals in the US Patent and Trademark Office has rejected the patent-drafting technique of defining a new *species* of micro-organism and claiming its use for the production of a new antibiotic, based on the disclosure of a number of *strains* having the common novel property of producing the antibiotic. The antibiotic, being new, was the subject of an allowed product claim. The main process claim which was rejected, however, was of the familiar 'circular' type in terms of a process for producing the designated antibiotic by culturing a micro-organism belonging to the newly named species (here *Micromonospora pilosospora*), the latter being defined in the claim as having the ability to produce the antibiotic. Three strains having this novel property had been discovered and deposited but the Board held that the disclosure of three strains was insufficient to enable the skilled person to locate a fourth strain having the same property. This argument is undoubtedly difficult to contest in many cases but its severity illustrates the typical difficulty of the microbiological inventor in extrapolating from his range of actual experimental results in order to secure adequately broad process protection. The applicant here was apparently concerned primarily with a point of principle, having obtained a claim to the antibiotic in the *per se* form which is generally regarded as the most effective form of patent protection.

Similarly in the United Kingdom the British Patent Office has rejected a new micro-organism species claim on the ground that the making available of a single strain, even if accompanied by an extensive description of its morphology and other properties, is insufficient to enable the skilled person to perform the invention across the range of a species claim. In this case the new species of micro-organism (*Micromonospora rosea* species *nova*) produced a known antibiotic thereby precluding a *per se* final product claim. There was therefore a strong motivation to protect the micro-organism itself in the broadest possible terms. However, it is difficult to achieve this on the basis of a single example, especially if the properties of the single isolate which are to be relied on as the definitive characteristics of the whole species are not clearly asserted to be such from the outset. It would then be necessary to establish that the skilled person would inevitably read this implication into the detailed description given for the specific strain deposited in the culture collection. It is noteworthy that the British Examiner had based himself on 'the established practice for microbiological inventions of this nature, which is to confine claims for novel micro-organisms and their use to what has actually been discovered and *not to permit the degree of predictive generalisation normally acceptable for chemical inventions*' (emphasis added).

There is therefore a definite imbalance between the microbiological and non-microbiological case which is magnified by the requirement to release a new micro-organism so early in the time-scale of patent procedure. Ideally the balance should in part be restored by postponing all availability of the deposited culture until the publication of an accepted patent application or grant of the corresponding patent takes place. This would harmonise with United States and Japanese practice and the long established national practice under the patent law of the Netherlands. Failing that, the independent expert solution should become available under national practices in harmony with that of the European patent system.

(v)   Use of the independent expert solution

Critics say that the independent expert solution has been little used. Even if few third parties avail themselves of the opportunity to nominate an independent expert to receive a sample of a deposited culture for investigation, a fair number of applicants do in fact opt for this alternative. One cannot assess the utility of this option simply by counting numbers. There will be many considerations to be taken into account in making decisions of this kind and these will always be unknown to official circles and indeed to any parties other than the applicants themselves. An applicant with an open licensing policy may use the independent expert option in the sensitive stages of negotiation but may in suitable cases desire the widest possible distribution of a deposited micro-organism from the earliest moment. Some applicants are refraining from using this solution in connection with European patent applications so long as hostility remains in some national official and legal circles in countries which are designated by the applicant for the European patent. Patenting in biotechnology is a predominantly international activity and there is little point in plugging a loophole in one's control of biological material in some countries so long as it has to be left open in others because of legal uncertainty or an unsympathetic official attitude.

(vi)   The necessity for reproducibility

Whereas a patent for a micro-organism *per se* can now be obtained in many countries on the basis of a timely deposit of the micro-organism in a culture collection, a few still insist on the necessity for a written description of a process for producing the micro-organism which is reproducible as a process in the hands of the skilled worker without resort to the deposited culture. In time this problem may wither away as regards certain kinds of microbiological invention. In the genetic engineering of micro-organisms, for example, more reliance may in future be placed on the ability of inventors to specify experimental methods with sufficient precision for the skilled worker to be enabled to reproduce the process for himself from the written description alone. For inventions involving the isolation of new micro-organisms from nature, however, the problem would appear to be a permanent one. It cannot be solved by the provision of a *total* description of the isolated strain, even where science can give one, because completeness of description of the organism does not alone guarantee access to it on the part of the reader if he has to re-isolate it for himself, as courts have already recognised.

5   **Legal protection for new plants**

There is a sharp contrast between United States patent law and European law in respect of the forms of protection available for plants produced either by traditional breeding processes or by modern genetic manipulation techniques. The US law permits virtually every possibility to be protected either by the utility patent or by the plant patent or by the certificate of protection, which latter corresponds to the plant variety right available elsewhere. Under US law the concept of the 'essentially biological' process as being outside the remit of patent protection is unknown. On the other hand Europe has created a dichotomy between the 'essentially biological' and the 'microbiological' which appears difficult to apply and stems entirely from the preconceived idea of separating the two areas of patent law and plant variety right law. This notional division no longer appears appropriate as the techniques of modern plant genetics develop.

(i)   Plant variety rights and patent protection

In Europe, the attempt to draw a legal line between microbiology and the 'higher' biology of plants and animals can be traced to a movement for unification of the patent laws of different countries which began with the so-called Strasbourg Convention of 1963 and saw its consummation for European countries in the European Patent Convention of 1973. This movement had been preceded by the UPOV Convention on plant variety rights and the patent legislators were convinced of the desirability of maintaining the separate system of plant variety protection without confusion or overlap with patent protection. Both the Strasbourg and European Conventions therefore excluded from patentability:

> 'plant or animal varieties or essentially biological processes for the production of plants or animals; this provision does not apply to microbiological processes or the products thereof.'

The UPOV Convention added its weight also to the desired dichotomy by providing that a member state having a patent law and a plant variety law could not offer both of them for the same botanical genus or species.

The fuzziness of the distinction between parts of biology was of no great practical concern over the decade or so following its introduction into the law. Plant breeders continued to utilise their own system which seems in general to have responded to the needs of commercial breeders and also of those in the public sector for all of whom the system of collecting royalties on manufacture and sale of propagating material gave a moderate return on the investment. Similarly, industrial microbiologists continued to work within the patent system and were sufficiently preoccupied with patent law problems which had arisen in what was indisputably their own area of technology. The legal professionals were equally focussed in their own respective fields especially in patent law where major changes had taken place during that time.

(ii)   The impact of plant biotechnology

· How will plant genetic manipulation impinge on the scene and what legal system will serve the interests of the innovators and entrepreneurs in this technology? It will be easier to answer this question when more case studies are to hand. It would be unfortunate, however, if and when commercially significant successes are achieved in the manipulation of plant genes to find that the laws available for protecting such inventions are inadequate for the purpose. We begin by asking how genetic manipulation will fit into the whole scheme for producing new or improved crop plants. Presumably such plants will not be 'zapped' into existence in the laboratory. The manipulative step may constitute only one part of the whole process of breeding a new variety and one which shortens the time taken by traditional breeding methods by introducing and distributing genetic variation more efficiently in the early stages. If this is so the system of rewarding the breeder by means of the licensing of plant variety rights may be the predominant mode of financial exploitation in which case the genetic manipulator may gain no more than a share of the financial return obtainable through this route. If the plant breeder deploys this expertise from within his organisation this consequence may not matter greatly because the cost is merged into the whole cost of the breeding programme. If, however, the genetic manipulation expertise comes from elsewhere and some return is expected by an independently funded source it is not immediately obvious how this sharing of the ultimate benefit would be structured. It is therefore desirable to see whether patent protection for genetic manipulation techniques and products would produce a different result.

For European patent law we can begin from the standpoint that genetic manipulation techniques of the kinds which have become well-known for procaryotes and the simpler eucaryotic systems are microbiological processes. On this there seems to be widespread agreement in official patent circles and therefore *inventive* methods of this kind are patentable. Under European patent law a patent for a process also covers the direct product of the process even if a formal claim to the product is not presented in the specification. The direct product of such a process will usually be the transformed plant cells and in such cases process claims to the technique and product claims covering the transformed cells will be obtainable. Where the patent disclosure also describes methods for regenerating new whole plants the applicant will almost certainly desire claims to the plants themselves in order to provide maximum coverage of all aspects of the invention in relation to commercial dealing up to and including the final marketed products. To take a hypothetical example, suppose it became possible to transfer a gene responsible for a certain pathogen-resistance in one plant (or other) species to a distant plant species or different plant genus, a patentee might well want to claim:

'Plants of the species (or genus) X having resistance to pathogens of the type Y by virtue of the transferred gene Z.'

The definitions of X and Y would need some thought as to the range of applicability of the inventive technique but probably more difficulty would attach to the selection of a definition for Z. To define Z in broad terms of gene function might be to claim too much whereas a definition in terms of a specific nucleotide sequence (assuming the knowledge was available) might be too narrow and easily avoidable.

To overcome the objection to granting patents for genetically modified plants it can be argued that the present law should be applicable only to new varieties produced by *conventional* plant breeding. Indeed, the justification for excluding plant varieties from patent protection is commonly stated in official circles to be the fact that legal protection is available by means of the plant variety right. This is true for varieties bred by the older methods. It must be observed, however, that this protection is essentially narrow in scope by being restricted precisely to the specific plant material subjected to the officially prescribed test procedures required in the assessment for plant variety protection (to establish distinctiveness, stability and homogeneity) and for official certification for commercial use. It does not cover generalised methods and techniques and more seriously, cannot cover a range of non-identical products, i.e. the protection is not generic. Inventive discoveries which lie ahead may well be of generic application and deserving of protection of the kind outlined in the exemplary patent claim given above. Such protection is at present inconceivable under any other form than patent protection.

By reflection upon the fundamental differences between the two types of right, official patent authorities may persuade themselves to interpret the exclusion from patent protection as narrowly as possible so as not to deny the proper form of protection to what in reality are inventions and not merely specific varieties. This has already been seen in a few countries and the signs are hopeful. Alternatively, one might seek to change the existing law so as to provide for an appropriate and effective type of patent protection. In either event, however, it would be necessary to show that a *reproducible* written description could be given which enabled these techniques to be repeated by persons skilled in the art.

Nevertheless, if patents were obtainable for plants appropriate methods of exploiting them are not immediately obvious to those whose experience is exclusively in the field of microbiological patents. Micro-organism patents in classical biotechnology do not call for extraordinary commercial measures in this respect. Thus in the majority of cases the development of new strains and their cultivation and use for the production of end products are all handled by or under the control of one commercial entity. There is nothing comparable to the breakdown of activities such as obtains in agricultural technology where we have the breeder, the seed merchant or nurseryman, and the growers between whom there are arms-length commercial transactions. The existence of plant patents of the kind described would introduce a new element into the agricultural and horticultural business and it is by no means clear what business mechanism the owners of such patents would choose to make their research efforts profitable. Although plant variety rights do not extend to consumption material, e.g. the plants themselves or their fruit, there is less reason under patent law why a plant patent owner should be debarred from securing a return on such material. It is perhaps principally for this reason that certain institutions are critical of any suggestion that existing plant variety law may not be well adapted to present day and foreseeable future developments in biotechnology affecting this industry.

6   Time-scale and the enforcement process

The problem of detecting and prohibiting secret infringement of process patents in biotechnology is virtually insoluble under present legal systems. The patentee is at an enormous disadvantage under this aspect of legal practice but there is no way out of this dilemma until the law recognises this fact. A patent granted after rigorous examination of the type current under European patent practice should be considered *prima facie* valid and enforceable and to justify the most generous application of the doctrine of the *prima facie* case to shift the burden of proof upon the alleged infringer. Furthermore under many national laws at present any attempt to enforce a patent will inevitably result in a counterclaim for a declaration of nullity or invalidity and this latter legal process seems to take preference over the infringement issue. Consequently there is delay in controlling unlawful commercial practices. This trend should be reversed and a balance restored. For example, if infringing activities were suspended pending the hearing of a genuine infringement suit the defendant would have an incentive to resolve the legal question rather than to delay its final outcome for as long as possible.

7   Awareness of patent law and the academic community

Such varied attitudes to the patent system as are shown by the international academic community are unsatisfactory and due to past misunderstandings which could be removed with mutual effort. Academic institutions should unhesitatingly accept that the patenting of academic inventions is worthwhile and is to be encouraged. A consensus among universities and similar institutions is desirable on this subject. It would also be helpful if some form of teaching on the basics of patent law were available for research workers in the faculties of natural sciences and technology such as by regular seminars to postgraduate students and by at least one or two lectures in every course of teaching for a first degree. The principles of ownership and responsibility for commercial exploitation of inventions arising in academic institutions should also be settled. As more institutions enter into research collaboration with industry, it may be useful for these institutions to have staff who are familiar with patent law and skilled in the exploitation (licensing) of industrial property. A small team of this kind need not operate to the exclusion of external sources of similar and even greater knowledge and experience in industrial property matters but could collaborate with them especially where there is external funding of the academic research.

For their part too, official patent circles should recognise the specific problems of the academic inventor and should invite representatives of academia to play a more active role in industrial property affairs. Academic involvement in the question of grace period provisions would be an obvious starting point in forging a link between the one world and the other.

Appendix 1: Glossary

Abandonment The act of allowing an application or patent to lapse by failure to take an action prescribed by law or regulation in order to maintain it. The action may be the filing of some document or of a response to an official action or the payment of a fee due within the prescribed period of time. Sometimes an application can be abandoned and refiled (see Refile).

Acceptance When official examination of a patent application is successfully completed the application is 'accepted'. Then, depending on local practice, the application may be laid open for possible Opposition by third parties or the patent may be granted.

Amendment This term signifies any change in an application or patent. Usually the change will be one of the text of the application or patent either in the claims or in the description. Amendment is most commonly carried out in response to objections from the Patent Office or from third parties in Opposition or other proceedings. An applicant or patentee may in suitable circumstances amend the application or patent voluntarily.

Application (patent) A formal application to a patent granting authority (Industrial Property Office, Patent Office) which involves the filing of formal documents prescribed by the appropriate law or official regulations including an 'Application form' or 'Request for grant' and a specification describing the invention. The terms 'application' and 'specification' are sometimes used synonymously.

Assignment The conveyance of ownership from one party to another. The term can apply to the process of transferring rights and also to the document of transfer, i.e. the assignment deed.

Budapest Convention (or Treaty) This Convention has the full title of 'The Budapest Treaty on the International Recognition of the Deposit of Micro-organisms for the Purposes of Patent Procedure'. It was established in April 1977 and came into force at the end of 1980. It provides for the recognition of culture collections as International Depositary Authorities (IDA) in any one of which a new strain of micro-organism can be deposited for the purposes of a patent application in

164

any member state. The following 22 states are members of this
Convention: Australia, Austria, Belgium, Bulgaria, Denmark, Finland,
France, Germany (Federal Republic), Hungary, Italy, Japan,
Liechtenstein, Netherlands, Norway, Philippines, Republic of Korea,
Soviet Union, Spain, Sweden, Switzerland, United Kingdom, United
States of America.

The following culture collections have IDA status:

> Agricultural Research Service Culture Collection, USA
> American Type Culture Collection, USA
> Centraalbureau voor Schimmelcultures, Netherlands
> Collection Nationale de Cultures de Micro-Organismes, France
> Culture Collection of Algae and Protozoa, UK
> Culture Collection of the CAB International Mycological
> Institute, UK
> Deutsche Sammlung von Mikroorganismen, Federal Republic
> of Germany
> European Collection of Animal Cell Cultures, UK
> Fermentation Research Institute, Japan
> In Vitro International Inc., USA
> Institute of Microoganism Biochemistry and Physiology of the
> USSR Academy of Science, Soviet Union
> National Bank for Industrial Microorganisms and Cell Cultures,
> Bulgaria
> Mezögazdasági és Ipari Mikroorganizmusok Magyar Nemzeti
> Gyüjteménye (National Collection of Agricultural and
> Industrial Microorganism), Hungary
> National Collection of Industrial Bacteria, UK
> National Collection of Type Cultures, UK
> National Collection of Yeast Cultures, UK
> USSR Research Institute for Antibiotics of the USSR Ministry
> of the Medical and Microbiological Industry, Soviet Union
> USSR Research Institute for Genetics and Industrial
> Microorganism Breeding of the USSR Ministry of the
> Medical and Microbiological Industry, Soviet Union

Case law Many principles of patent law are stated explicitly in written
statutes. Others are derived from decisions of courts of law in particular
cases and these are referred to collectively as case law. Case law is
binding or at least influential on subsequent decisions of Courts at the
same or lower level. From time to time established case law becomes
codified into written statutes when new or amending legislation occurs.
As regards biotechnology a considerable body of precedent now exists
in the form of case law.

Citation A document cited as prior art by a Patent Office Examiner in an official action or by a third party in Opposition or other contentious proceeding.

Claims The claims of an application or patent are verbal formulae defining the invention or the scope of protection sought or obtained. These are appended to the technical description and together therewith form the specification as a whole. Claims are expressed in process, product, or other appropriate form. (See also 'Product claims.')

Conception In US patent practice conception means the mental act creating the invention. Conception is established when the first documentary record is made of the idea, even before any laboratory experiments have been carried out. To be effective towards establishing an 'invention date' this record must be made in or introduced into the USA.

Continuation In USA (only) an application can be followed by a 'continuation' application which reproduces the total original disclosure. This kind of application is called a 'file wrapper continuation' (FWC) because the contents of the official file of the original application are transferred or copied to the file of the continuation application. The FWC must be lodged before abandoning its predecessor and it is then entitled, for priority purposes, to the date of its predecessor. The filing of FWC applications can be used to obtain further time in which to produce an effective response to official objections, should the normal period of time allowed for this purpose be insufficient. The filing of such applications can apparently be repeated many times.

Continuation-in-part (CIP) In USA this is a special type of continuation application and differs from the FWC application in that it contains matter additional to what is disclosed in its predecessor (parent) application. It must also be filed before abandonment of the parent application and is entitled, for priority purposes, to the parent application date for common subject matter, i.e. disclosed in the parent as well as in the CIP. The additional material takes its own filing date for priority purposes. This is apparently a highly useful facility when research is continually and rapidly developing, allowing updating of the specification to provide the strongest disclosure. However its use must be carefully considered especially where publication of the original specification, e.g. in the form of its counterparts in other countries, or where academic or other publication of the original invention has occurred in the meantime. The US attorney is the only person fully competent to advise on the use of CIP applications in specific circumstances.

Deposit of micro-organisms in culture collections The primary function of culture collections is to accept the deposit of strains of micro-organism from scientific workers as a service to the scientific community, providing an authoritative source of reference and supply of particular micro-organisms for use in scientific research and in industry. In recent years the lodging of new strains with culture collections for purposes connected with patent applications (sometimes described as 'patent cultures') has become established as a necessary or desirable procedure in order to support the written description of the micro-organism in the corresponding patent application. Deposited strains are allotted accession dates and accession numbers by which they are identified and referred to in the patent specification.

Division Division, or 'dividing out', is the act of separating a patent application into two or more applications. The original application is the parent application and the new application is the divisional application. The claims of a divisional application are entitled to the priority date of the parent application for subject matter which is disclosed therein.

European Patent Convention (EPC) Established in October 1973 and coming into force in June 1978 this Convention provides for a single patent application to be prosecuted before the European Patent Office (EPO) designating any number of contracting states. The initial application may be made in any of the regional offices of the EPO (national Patent Offices) but is in due course examined by the EPO in Munich. Upon grant the European patent does not mature into a single item of property but enters the national phase in each designated state and emerges as a 'bundle' of national patents, e.g. European patent (UK), European patent (France) etc. which thereafter become independent objects of property. At present the following 13 states are parties to this Convention: Austria, Belgium, France, Germany (Federal Republic), Greece, Italy, Liechtenstein, Luxembourg, Netherlands, Spain, Sweden, Switzerland, United Kingdom.

Under the Community Patent Convention (not yet in operation) a single application filed through the European Patent Office will mature into a single unitary indivisible object of property covering the whole of the European Economic Community.

Grace period The all-embracing definition of the state of the art in the Strasbourg and European Patent Conventions has been adopted in many national patent laws in European countries as part of the policy of harmonisation with European law. As a result this has eliminated from some national laws previous provisions exempting from the general rule of novelty any publication emanating from the applicant himself. These publications were not prejudicial to the applicant's position provided a patent application was filed within a specific period and this came to be known as a 'grace period'. The United Kingdom and Germany previously allowed a grace period of six months. The United States and

Canada have even longer grace periods and these are still part of their national law. (See Appendix 4.)

National patents These are granted according to the laws of individual States and have effect only within the jurisdiction of the relevant State. In the field of patent law, however, there is a strong tradition of over a century of international co-operation by means of International Conventions which regulate formal and substantive patent matters between member States.

Official Action A report is issued by a Patent Office Examiner on the result of his examination of a patent application. The report may cite prior art found by the Examiner and may also contain other objections to the specification and claims and also to formal matters. In most countries a reply to the official action must be filed within the specified term, which can sometimes be extended on payment of an additional fee, otherwise the application will be officially treated as abandoned. In most countries such abandonment is irretrievable but in some the application may be resuscitated, again with a fee penalty.

Opposition The grant of a patent may be opposed by an interested party if he can raise objections which comply with the grounds of Opposition prescribed by law. Under the European patent system formal Opposition may be filed within nine months of the grant of the European patent. In Japan and some other countries Opposition is filed before the formal grant of patent rights and in a prescribed period following final publication of the accepted application. United States and Canada do not provide for Opposition. In the UK the procedure which corresponds to European Opposition is termed 'Revocation'.

Paris Convention This has the full title of 'The International Convention for the Protection of Industrial Property' and was founded in 1883. The member States which have ratified this convention (and which are sometimes described as members of the Paris Union) now number 97 states and include the great majority of the industrialised world. Member States must treat nationals of other member States of the Union equally with their own nationals as regards the protection of industrial property. One of the most important articles of the Paris Convention recognises the first filing of a patent application in any member State as establishing a right of priority, as of its filing date, which will also be accorded to a corresponding patent application in any other member State if the latter is filed within 12 months of the first filing. The text of the Paris Convention has been modified several times, the latest being the Stockholm text of 1967.

Product claims These are of two main types, the product *per se* claim and the product-by-process claim. A *per se* claim is one that extends to the substance or micro-organism as such and is independent of any defined process of preparation or derivation. This is also referred to as absolute product protection. A product-by-process claim, on the other hand, defines a substance or micro-organism in terms of some particular method of production. Hence it is more limited in scope as compared with the *per se* claim and is avoided by the choice of a method or route to the procurement of the product different from that defined in the claim.

A form of product claim is sometimes met which uses process terminology to indicate how the product may be obtained but which does not restrict the claim to the use of such a process; though apparently in product-by-process form such a claim is in reality a product *per se* claim.

Reduction in practice As with conception the term 'reduction to practice' is used in the parlance of US patent law. It signifies the translation of an inventive concept into an operational process, model or prototype of an invention. This is known as actual reduction to practice. Also as for conception, reduction to practice must take place in the USA to be effective in establishing invention date for the purposes of US patent law.

Refile An application can be abandoned and replaced by another application covering the same subject matter or the same with additional matter, either immediately following the abandonment or soon after. The 'refiled' application cannot benefit from the date of the original application and must take its own filing date for priority purposes. Refiling after abandonment is therefore a ploy to 'restart the clock' as far as all aspects of patent procedure are concerned. It can only be done in the absence of publication of the invention before the filing date of the new application. 'Abandon and refile' tactics are a device for starting the process afresh based on a new priority date and must therefore be distinguished from the continuation applications filed under US practice which preserve the original effective date.

Renewal fees In most countries the maintaining of a patent is subject to the payment of renewal fees which are usually required annually. US patents granted on applications filed before 12 December 1980 do not require the payment of renewal fees but those granted on applications filed after this date have renewal fees payable at prescribed times.

Specification (patent) The written description of an invention which must be filed when an application for a patent is made. This must include a technical description which can be appreciated by a person of ordinary skill in the art concerned and a statement (one or more 'claims') of the scope of protection sought. The term 'patent' is often used to denote the specification but this usage is only strictly correct after the grant of patent rights.

Strasbourg Convention This is the 'Convention on the Unification of
Certain Points of Substantive Law on Patents for Invention' and dates
from November 1963. Many of the features of this convention have been
incorporated into the European Patent Convention, notably the
definition of the 'state of the art' against which the degree of novelty
and inventiveness of the subject matter of a patent application must be
judged.

State of the art In the language of patent law this expression is used in a
somewhat different sense to that which it has in science and technology.
In the European Patent Convention the state of the art is defined as

> 'Everything made available to the public by means of a written
> or oral description, by use, or in any other way, before the date
> of filing of the European patent application.'

The above definition signifies all that is part of public knowledge and
experience before the attempt is made to protect an invention. Thus it is
another form of reference to the prior art, i.e. that which is old and
therefore cannot be patented.

Appendix 2: Copyright and DNA

The idea that DNA sequences and other biologically significant products constructed by the molecular biologist can be the subject of copyright protection is an intriguing one. It has been proposed by a few commentators, mostly in the USA, but majority opinion considers it to be flawed both in theory and practice. Many lawyers reject the argument out of hand as not deserving of legal analysis but the wide language of copyright law, especially United States law, can be made to read very easily on many biological events and it is instructive to seek out the fallacy in the argument if such there be.

Copyright law either in written statutory form or as interpreted by the courts forbids the copying or reproduction in physical form of a 'copyright work' created by an 'author'. The forbidden activities include all the known ways by hand or machine of creating one or more copies of the original work without the permission of the copyright author or owner. In the application of genetic engineering methods the manipulator is using the machinery of living cells to reproduce DNA sequences, recombinant plasmids, transformed micro-organisms and other entities.

Copyright law is mainly concerned with the protection of literary and artistic creations and works of artistic craftsmanship. All of these come under the general description of 'works of authorship'. The first question must therefore be whether the chemical products and biological systems created by chemical and biochemical processes can be said to be the kinds of thing contemplated as works of authorship in the law of copyright. Before answering this question it should be noted that engineering drawings have long been held to qualify for copyright protection. Drawings are literary works. Copyright is therefore not restricted to what most people would class as artistic works. Moreover it is now widely accepted that computer programs and data bases can be the subject of copyright; these are literary works which can be expressed and fixed in tangible form on cards or tapes and then 'read' by machine. A most impressive analogy can be made between the information which is stored in and conveyed electronically by computer programs and the biological 'information' which is contained in a DNA sequence fixed in the tangible form of a plasmid or chromosome and which is read by the enzymatic machinery of the cell involved in protein synthesis.

171

The argument for the relevance of copyright to the products and processes of genetic engineering is based essentially on legal theory and skilful application to the context of copyright law of the metaphorical terms used to describe biological events and systems e.g. copying, reproduction, information, expression, gene libraries and so on. The contrary theoretical argument is that DNA sequences, plasmids, and living cells are not works of authorship within the meaning of copyright law and that a court would reject such a far-fetched interpretation of this term.

From the practical viewpoint the copyright argument becomes even more difficult to sustain. In a legal action for infringement of copyright, actual copying of the author's work must be shown or clearly inferred from the circumstances. The word 'copying' here carries not only its legal meaning of reproduction but also the moral aspect of imitation or plagiarism. Usually the defendant has seen the success of the plaintiff's product and has copied it, in the latter sense, by making one just like it. It can be inferred that the defendant has not independently created his own design and cannot therefore rebut the charge of copying. In these circumstances the copying of the plaintiff's product will be held to infringe the copyright in the original drawing, the copyright work, of the author.

Now in order to establish infringement of a patent it is not necessary for a court to have actual proof of copying or reach the conclusion that there was a deliberate intention to copy the patentee's marketed product. The test for patent infringement is whether the defendant's product falls within the scope of the patent claims. If it does, the question of intention is unimportant on the main issue although it can affect the level of damages payable to the patentee. Moreover there is no escape from the charge of infringement by demonstrating independent discovery in the defendant's research laboratory. Even *prior* discovery by the defendant will not be a defence in a patent infringement action. When the question of proof of copyright infringement is considered in biotechnology situations it becomes difficult to see how one would proceeed in a practical case. The infringer would have to be shown at least to have had access to the recombinant plasmid or recombinant strain which he is alleged to have copied.

Finally it must be pointed out that copyright is a narrow form of protection. It does not protect an underlying idea but only the form in which that idea is expressed by the copyright author (in theatrical terms it can cover the script but not the plot). In genetic manipulation therefore there could be considerable room for evasion of copyright if copyright were applicable at all to products of the kind in question. The reader must therefore suspend judgement on this ingenious idea and not regard it as any short cut to obtaining protection in this field.

Appendix 3: Patents and trade secrecy

Valuable discoveries made in the research laboratory can be published, patented or held in secret. These three options are not in all cases completely incompatible, however, and a careful blend of policies is sometimes possible. We have seen in Chapter 2 and subsequent chapters that a policy of rapid publication of research findings as and when they arise is the only one that cannot be made to work in harmony with the others. Whilst it may be good for the purposes of academic record, the serial publication of incremental developments in a line of research without benefit of patent protection makes it virtually impossible to control the commercial utilisation of this knowledge.

The principal alternatives to be considered here are those of patenting versus secrecy. The common term used for the latter is 'trade secrecy' but its meaning is not limited to trading alone. Trade secrets are not the subject of statutes of the kind that exist for patents, designs and trade marks and it is arguable whether they should be classed as intellectual property as such. Disputes over trade secrets in the Anglo-Saxon legal tradition come under the common law and various definitions of what constitute trade secrets have been given by the courts from time to time. Almost anything that is a secret and gives its owners a competitive advantage can be held to be a trade secret. Trade secrets therefore cover a much wider range than invention or innovation and extend to commercial information of all kinds, e.g. a confidential list of a firm's customers. For comparative purposes, the availability of trade secret protection must take into account inventions that could otherwise be the subject of patent protection as well as the corresponding know-how which cannot normally be dealt with by means of patents.

The main reason that patents and trade secrets are at opposite poles is that publication is the inevitable result of patenting and indeed is an important part and justification of the patent system. In modern patent practice publication of the contents of patent applications has been brought forward to such an early stage in patent procedure that the 'lead time' an inventor can enjoy before information about his invention becomes public is now reduced to an insignificant amount. Historically publication was a consequence of official acceptance of a patent application or the actual grant of patent rights. Now, however, publication takes place in many countries irrespective of whether or not rights will be granted and long before the applicant can fully assess his chances of obtaining useful claims. The disadvantages of this feature of early publication are most acute in the case of microbiological inventions (see Chapter 6). Also once the Patent Office have completed preparations to publish the application there is no turning back in order to avoid it. The inventor or his employer must therefore make the choice between patenting and secrecy as soon as an invention has reached the stage of development at which it can be evaluated for patent protection. If knowledge of an invention will inevitably come into the public domain either because the inventor feels compelled to write a paper or otherwise disclose it so that it can be repeated by other workers, or because commercial activities will have much the same effect, then patenting is obviously the only choice if any protection is to be had.

Where a true choice exists as between patenting and secrecy the main factors involved are as follows.

1   Scope and effectiveness of patent protection

Where it is expected that strong and broad patent claims will issue which will adequately protect a product to be put on the market or a process to be used for this purpose, and will also protect against modifications so that the patent will not be easy to avoid by competitors, there will be a strong case for seeking patent protection. Where a substantial investment in research has been required to develop the product to the marketing stage then patents will be of particular importance especially if competitors are likely to make the same invention independently. If the product or process can be readily 'reverse engineered' from an examination of the product or from any information which becomes available about it, patenting must be a preferred option. Where the patent is of a kind which enables its owner to maintain exclusivity for a sufficient period and consequently to secure a major share of the market, this consequence may continue even after the patent has expired. The strongest position from this point of view must be one in which adequately broad product claims not limited to any particular process or manufacture can be obtained. However even where only process protection is available the value of patent protection should not be discounted as important process patents are necessary as part of a total strategy of building patent strength.

To make a proper assessment of the patent position it will be necessary to have carried out the best possible search of the prior art. If such a search has revealed a fair amount of close prior art which will make it almost impossible to obtain protection for anything other than marginal differences it would be appropriate to reject the patent route for fear of disclosing too much information which could be useful to competitors.

2 Enforceability of the protection

If a patent cannot readily be policed or enforced its publication will merely alert others to the invention and its potential. If other parties are confident that the risks of being sued are small some may be tempted to make use of the disclosure and practise the invention in the hope that they will not be found out and sued. Enforceability of a patent therefore depends upon (1) detection of infringement and (2) providing proof of infringement. In general there is a major distinction here as between a product patent and a process patent. A product patent containing a *per se* claim to the substance or other product will give the strongest position because the appearance of the infringing product on the market will itself provide the evidence of infringement. With a process patent proof of infringement may be feasible if an analysis of the product will reveal the process used in its manufacture. Alternatively there may be no other known way of making the particular product than by the patented process. In all these cases the patentee can proceed if he can show a *prima facie* case of infringement whereupon formal proof may be obtained later by actual inspection of the process used by the other party.

If the invention can be given only limited patent protection, involving difficult policing and enforcement problems, trade secrecy will be the preferred option. This is especially the case for minor process improvements for the manufacture of known products where the detection of infringement would be extremely difficult. However there are situations in which even though use of a process invention cannot be revealed by careful analysis of the marketed product the invention has a high intrinsic value and importance and there is a high probability that the same invention will be made independently by others. In such a situation the initial investment in research effort deserves patent protection to protect this investment.

A great deal of uncertainty attaches to the enforceability of the vast majority of patents and the difficulty even for the most seasoned patent lawyers to predict the outcome is a definite drawback of following the patent route. Some of this uncertainty can be eliminated by the most thorough searching of the prior art either before a patent application is first filed or later during prosecution and certainly before litigation is commenced. It is an unfortunate fact however that even though the applicant has searched diligently and various Patent Offices have also cited what they consider to be relevant prior art, it cannot safely be assumed that an exhaustive knowledge is thereby gained. Frequently a defendant in a patent infringement suit will have been able to unearth more prior art that has a bearing on the issues of novelty and inventiveness and which introduces the element of surprise.

3   Cost of enforcement and time-scales

The greatest routine cost of following the patent route derives from the large number of countries in which protection is often required. The choice of a foreign filing programme is one of the most difficult decisions to be made in the lifetime of any patent situation and there are no short cuts. Sometimes the true potential worth of an invention is not realised until years after this decision has had to be made and one can find in retrospect that the amount of territorial cover obtained has been too small. The major companies have their strategies for dealing with this problem depending on the nature of the invention, whether it be product or process, and where manufacture of the product might take place. So long as the major manufacturing countries are protected it may be possible to leave some small countries uncovered, relying on a possible infringement suit in a manufacturing country to prevent exportation to the unprotected user country.

These routine costs which cover the official fees to be paid and the professional services involved in prosecuting the patent applications to grant are dwarfed by the high cost of enforcement by litigation. Fortunately far more patents are obtained than ever come into court and many of them are not challenged. The high cost of litigation is a major problem for the small company which wishes to hold patents and have them respected by larger competitors. Whether a patent is to be enforced or not is nevertheless a commercial decision which must take into account many factors. The likelihood of winning or losing is probably the first essential question to be considered. Even when a conclusion has been reached on this however the market size must always justify the cost of enforcement. The time factor is also crucial in any technology in which inventions become obsolete after a relatively few years. It is almost impossible to obtain a patent in any of the important examining countries in less than two or three years and this period can often be prolonged by the action taken by the competitors to oppose the grant of the patent. Litigation also takes many years to conclude. How much life there will be left in the patent or how much commercial life there will be left in the product at the end of the whole patenting and litigation process will affect the decision to litigate or not.

4   The protection conferred by secrecy

Some trade secrets have remained secret long after a patent would have expired. The combination of a secret process and a very good trade mark is a very formidable one for a patent to beat and its owner can reap commercial benefit almost indefinitely. Two of the most frequently cited examples of this are the product sold under the trade mark 'Coca-Cola' and the even older secret formula for 'Chartreuse' liqueur to the makers of which a commitment to perpetual silence is not uncongenial!

The protection given by secrecy depends entirely on the maintenance of secrecy. Once a secret is breached the available legal remedies lie against the person disclosing the secret. Once the secret is out however there is little that can be done to put the clock back and it will rarely be possible to recover in damages sufficient compensation from the person who has betrayed the confidence. The feasibility of maintaining a trade secret by compartmentalising the information so that no one member of staff knows of a significant portion of the process will depend entirely on the circumstances. The costs of establishing and maintaining elaborate security precautions of this kind may also be substantial.

5   Protectionist or licensing policies

Trade secrecy is more easy to reconcile with a wholly protectionist policy on behalf of a company or individual opposed to the basic idea of technology transfer. Secret processes and know-how can of course be the subject of licence agreements but there is a limit to the scale on which licensing can be carried out in these circumstances whilst at the same time maintaining effective control over the secret nature of the data and information. In general patents are more convenient instruments of technology transfer by licensing because the scope of the agreement and the field of the agreement are usually controlled by the patent situation. Disputes between licensor and licensee can arise in which the licensee claims that he is operating outside the scope of the licensed patents, at least over part of his manufacturing activities, and the matter can be settled by reference to the patent claims. This pre-supposes that the relationship is one of a straight patent licence rather than a mixed licence (which admittedly is much more common) covering patent rights and know-how in which case some know-how may be utilised by the licensee even though he has moved outside the strict scope of the licensed patents. Stated another way, a patent constitutes a tangible and precise claim to an invention whereas in a know-how agreement there may be some doubt as to the relevance of the transferred data and information to the commercial activities of the licensee.

The brief analysis given above of the factors to be considered in making the choice between patent protection and secrecy covers the most salient and simple elements. In practice the problem will often be a highly complex one involving a careful balance of opposing considerations. The insights of inventors, patent advisers, and the commercial business arm of any industrial company or other organisation may all be necessary to reach the correct decision.

Appendix 4: Grace periods

A 'grace period' is a period of time before the filing of a patent application in which certain types of public disclosure or use of an invention described in the patent application will not prevent a valid patent being granted on the application. To qualify for benefit of a grace period the disclosure or use must be traceable to knowledge originating from the applicant or a person connected with the applicant by a chain of legal ownership or some other special relationship, e.g. the inventor or a predecessor in title of the applicant. It does not apply therefore to a disclosure deriving from any other person who has generated the information independently.

The term 'grace period' can be used in relation to disclosures made either with or without the consent of the applicant or connected person. The first of these alternatives corresponds more exactly with the primary meaning of the term which conveys the idea of a favour or pardon excusing someone from the consequences of a 'fault' committed. In relation to the second alternative the term 'grace' is being used somewhat artificially since the applicant is by hypothesis 'innocent' of the offending disclosure which is against his interest. Disclosures made without the applicant's consent are sometimes made through breach of confidence arising from a genuine mistake or misunderstanding or for some other reason.

The term 'grace period' is also often applied to the exemption given in some laws, e.g. the European Patent Convention, for disclosures made at officially recognised Exhibitions within six months before the filing of the application. Since such cases are rare they will not figure in the following discussion. The real issue with regard to grace periods is whether or not the patent law should protect inventors from the consequences of their deliberate public disclosures and what should be the extent of any such protection if it is to be allowed. Examples of grace period provisions which already exist in patent law are shown in Table A4.1. With regard to the type of disclosure the column headed 'abuse' refers to breach of confidence situations while the heading 'academic publication' is shorthand for disclosures at scientific meetings and in learned society publications. The precise nature of the protected disclosures in the latter case should be carefully checked against local law. The length of the grace period is the period preceding the actual

179

Table A4.1 *Grace period provisions*

Country	Type of disclosure			Grace period
	any	abuse	academic	
USA	✓			1 year
Canada	✓			2 years*
EPC		✓		6 months
European national		✓		6 months
Portugal			✓	1 year
Brazil			✓	1 year
Japan			✓	6 months
Australia } New Zealand }			✓	6 months

* Recently changed to 1 year

filing date in the particular country or legal system concerned and does not relate to priority date. Some of the arguments for and against the principle of a grace period are as follows.

Arguments in favour

1. Through ignorance of the law an inventor may through preliminary disclosure destroy his chances of obtaining protection.
2. An inventor may fail to recognise that an important invention has been made until after it has been disclosed to others.
3. The importance of information flow among the research community is paramount. A grace period would encourage dissemination of information, would avoid mistrust between scientists and other persons and would recognise the fact that academic publication is often the first disclosure of important new research discoveries.
4. Inventors often need to collaborate with others in the development of their invention. For example an invention may have to be disclosed to others for purposes of testing or in the course of testing.
5. A grace period would prevent the over-hasty filing of patent applications on incomplete inventions and thereby relieve some of the burden on patent examining authorities.
6. It is often difficult for individual inventors or small firms to maintain the level of secrecy required by the patent law. The

leakage of information may occur in a way which is not easily brought within the terms of an 'evident abuse' of the inventor's or applicant's rights.

Arguments against

1. The absolute novelty principle is easy to understand and makes for legal clarity.
2. A grace period creates legal doubt for third parties as regards the state of the art, particularly with regard to written publications and products on the market.
3. Inventors should be induced to file patent applications without undue delay in view of the informational function of the patent system.
4. A grace period would induce in inventors a false sense of security and would not protect them from intervening disclosures made by third parties.
5. A grace period extends the effective period of protection beyond the term allowed by patent law.
6. A grace period is of interest and value only to a minority of inventors.

Appendix 5: European Patent Office Guidelines on Rule 28

1. Specific comments on the relevant information on the characteristics of the most important groups of microorganisms

1.1 Bacteria

Standard literature: R.E. Buchanan, N.E. Gibbons: Bergey's Manual of Determinative Bacteriology.

Characterisation:

When classifying a bacterium strain under a known species, use of the criteria laid down in Bergey's Manual and of any other specific morphological or physiological peculiarity is recommended. When describing a **new** species, genus can first be determined as per Bergey and subsequently a comparison made with known species. The significant criteria vary from one group of bacteria to another.

Typical standard media are:

– Brain Heart Infusion, e.g. BBI No. 01-256
– Trypton Soy Broth, e.g. Oxoid No. CM 129
– Nutrient Agar

1.2 Actinomycetes

Characterisation:

As for bacteria.

Typical standard media:

– Bacto Actinomycete Isolation Agar, e.g. Difco No. 0957
– Tryptone Soy Broth, e.g. Oxoid No. CM 129
– Yeast Extract/Malt Extract Agar
– Oatmeal Agar
– Inorganic Salts/Starch Agar

1.3 Yeasts

Standard literature: J. Lodder & N.J.W. Kreger van Rij: The Yeast, a Taxonomic Study.

Characterisation:

As the morphology is usually little differentiated, the physiology is more significant for differentiation purposes. Description of known and new yeast species as for bacteria.

Typical standard media:

– Yeast Extract Agar, e.g. Oxoid No. CM 19
– Czapek Dox Medium, e.g. Difco No. B 338
– Malt Extract Agar
– Peptone Dextrose Agar

1.4 Fungi

Standard Literature: G.C. Ainsworth, F.K. Sparrow, A.S. Sussman: The Fungi.

April 1983

In addition, special monographs on particular fungus genera, e.g. J.J. Pitt: The Genus Penicillium.

Characterisation:

Initial differentiation on the basis of morphology, more specific differentiation on the basis of physiology. Description of known and new fungus species as for bacteria.

Typical standard media:

– Yeast Extract Agar, e.g. Oxoid No. CM 19
– Czapek Dox Medium, e.g. Difco No. B 338
– Potato Dextrose Agar

2. Typical characterisation data

Bearing the above in mind, the characterisation data "relevant" for the purposes of Rule 28, paragraph (1)(b) can be found among the following parameters.

2.1 Morphological characteristics (for bacteria: e.g. size and shape of vegetative cells, size, shape and number of spores, motility, gram-staining; for actionomycetes, yeasts and fungi: e.g. size and shape of vegetative cells, hyphae, mycelia, size, shape and number of spores) on suitable media.

2.2 Physiology and growth (including growth conditions such as pH, aeration requirement and temperature) on suitable media – cf. the above recommendations – also minimal medium; indication of characteristic features observed under those conditions (e.g. colour; shape, gloss, pigment on agar media; growth characteristics in liquid media) and

– assimilation, (e.g. nitrate, different C-sources)

– requirement, (N-sources, C-sources, energy sources, vitamins, amino acids etc.) of organic and inorganic materials

– decomposition, and/or
– production
– products of metabolism

2.3 Taxonomic classification as per the keys given in the standard literature referred to above.

2.4 Process for the production of mutants, plasmids, etc.

Appendix 6: Japanese Patent Office Informal Guidelines for examination of inventions relating to genetic engineering as received from Japanese patent attorneys

PREFACE

When an invention relating to genetic engineering is examined, the guidelines for examination of inventions relating to "applied microbial industry" and "microorganism *per se*", which have been published, will be applied to the examination of an invention relating to genetic engineering, so long as the invention is concerned with a microorganism.

1. *INDUSTRIAL FIELDS*

These guidelines are applied to an invention relating to genetic engineering among those relating to a microorganism.

Note 1: "Microorganism" means yeast, mold, fungus, bacterium, actinomycetes, unicellular algae, virus, protist and the like, and further includes cells of animal and plant.

Note 2: "Genetic engineering" means the techniques by which genes are artifically manipulated, such as gene recombination and cell fusion.

Note 3: "Invention relating to a microorganism" includes inventions of foreign genes, vectors or recombinant vectors *per se*, which are prepared by or from or introduced into microorganism.

2. *DEPOSITION OF MICROORGANISM*

(1) *TRANSFORMANT*

A.   In an invention relating to a transformant created from a microorganism by the gene recombinant technique, when the creation process of the transformant can be fully described in the specification so that an ordinary skilled person in the technical field with which the invention is concerned (hereinafter referred to as "a skilled person in the art") can reproduce the transformant, the creation process must be described in the originally filed specification, while the microorganism used for the creation of the transformant must be deposited to any depositary organization designated by the Director General of the Patent Office (PTO) or any international depositary authority referred to in Article 2 (viii) of Budapest Treaty on the International Recognition of the Deposit of Microorganisms for the Purposes of Patent Procedure, and the accession number given to the microorganism must be described in the originally filed specification, with the exception where the microorganism can be readily available to a skilled person in the art.

B.   In an invention relating to a transformant, when it is difficult to describe the creation process of the transformant in the specification so that a skilled person in the art can reproduce the transformant, the transformant must be deposited and its accession number must be described in the originally filed specification.

(2) *FOREIGN GENE, VECTOR AND RECOMBINANT VECTOR*

A.   In an invention relating to a foreign gene, a vector or a recombinant vector which is prepared by or from a microorganism, the preparation process thereof must be described in the originally filed specification so that a skilled person in the art can reproduce the foreign gene, vector or recombinant vector while, when the micro-organism used for the preparation thereof can not readily be available to a skilled person in the art, the micro-organism must be deposited and its accession number must be described in the originally filed specification.

B.   In an invention relating to a foreign gene, a vector or a recombinant vector, when it is difficult to describe the preparation process thereof in the specification so that a skilled person in the art can reproduce the foreign gene, vector or recombinant vector, a microorganism into which the foreign gene, vector or recombinant vector prepared has been introduced may be deposited and its accession number may be described in the originally filed specification, so that the means for providing the foreign gene, vector or recombinant vector prepared can be clarified.

(3) *PREPARATION METHOD OF FOREIGN GENE, VECTOR, RECOMBINANT VECTOR OR TRANSFORMANT*

In an invention relating to a method of preparation of a foreign gene, a vector, a recombinant vector or a transformant, the preparation process thereof must be described in the originally filed specification so that a skilled person in the art can perform the preparation procedures while, when the microorganism used for the preparation procedures can not readily be available to a skilled person in the art, the microorganism must be deposited and its accession number must be described in the originally filed specification.

(4) *PREPARATION METHOD OF CHEMICAL SUBSTANCES BY USE OF TRANSFORMANT*

In an invention relating to a method of preparation of a chemical substance or the like with the use of a transformant, when the transformant used can not readily be available to a skilled person in the art, the means for obtaining the transformant must be clearly described in the originally filed specification according to (1) A or B.

3. *UTILITY*

In an invention relating to a foreign gene, a vector, a recombinant vector, a transformant or a fused cell, their utility (usefulness) must be described with some reliability in the originally filed specification.

4. *DESCRIPTION (SPECIFICATION AND CLAIMS)*

(1) *CLAIMS*

A. *FOREIGN GENE*

(i)   A foreign gene should be defined in principle by the base sequence (nucleotide sequence).

[Example] Human interferon gene having the base sequence: TGTGAT......AAGGAA.

(ii)   When an amino acid sequence coded by the base sequence of a foreign gene is novel, the foreign gene can be defined by the amino acid sequence, even if the illustrated base sequence in the specification is only one example.

[Note] A base sequence encoding for an amino acid sequence generally has some degeneracies.

[Example] Human interferon gene encoding for the amino acid sequence: MetAsp......LysGlu.

(iii)   When a foreign gene can not be specifically defined by its base sequence, such a foreign gene may be defined by a specific combination of the functions, physicochemical properties, source of origin from which the gene is derived, the preparation method and the like of the gene. However, a definition of a foreign gene by its function(s) only can not be accepted in principle.

B. *VECTOR*

A vector is defined by its DNA base sequence or by a combination of its cleavage map (restriction map), molecular weight and/or number of base pairs, source of origin and/or preparation method, functions and/or properties which characterize the vector, and the like.

C. *RECOMBINANT VECTOR*

A recombinant vector is defined by a combination of a foreign gene as defined in (1) A and a vector as defined in (1) B.

If either the foreign gene or the vector is not limited to the specific one, such a recombinant vector can be defined by either the foreign gene or the vector only.

[Example] A vector containing DNA having the following base sequence: ACAGCA......AGTCAC.

D. *TRANSFORMANT*

A transformant is defined by a combination of a host microorganism expressed by the name of a strain with the name of species or genus in accordance with the microbial nomenclature and a recombinant vector.

If the host microorganism is not limited to the specific species, such a host microorganism can be described by a range of microorganisms extending the specific species which should be reasonable in accordance with the disclosure of the specification.

E. *FUSED CELL*

A fused cell is defined by a combination of a parent cell used and the functions, properties, preparation method and the like of the fused cell.

(2) *SPECIFICATION (DETAILED DESCRIPTION OF THE INVENTION)*

A. *FOREIGN GENE, VECTOR AND RECOMBINANT VECTOR*

In an invention relating to a foreign gene, a vector or a recombinant vector, the specification must describe the definition, the functions and properties, the method of preparation and, if necessary, the embodiments (examples) of the claimed foreign gene, vector or recombinant vector.

(i)   The functions and properties must be described objectively and substantially and, if necessary, with experimental data, etc.

(ii)   The method of preparation includes the source of origin, utilized enzymes, treatment conditions, recovery and purification processes, identification methods, etc.

B. *TRANSFORMANT*

In an invention relating to a transformant, the definition, the functions and properties, the method of preparation and, if necessary, the embodiments (examples) of the claimed transformant.

(i)   The functions and properties must be described objectively and substantially and, if necessary, with experimental data, etc.

(ii)   The method of preparation includes the recombinant vector, the host microorganism, the method of introduction of the recombinant vector, the methods of selection and recovery of the transformant, the means for identification and the like.

C. *FUSED CELL*

In an invention relating to a fused cell, a parent cell, the functions and properties, the preparation method and the like must be definitely described.

The method of preparation of the fused cell includes the pretreatment of the parent cell, the fusion conditions, the methods of selection and recovery of the fused cell, the methods of identification and the like.

Appendix 7: Suggestions for further reading

Introductory books

Patents in Chemistry and Biotechnology, P. W. Grubb, 2nd edition, Clarendon Press, Oxford, 1986.
Patenting in the Biological Sciences, R. S. Crespi, John Wiley & Sons, 1982, Chichester.

Yeasts: Living Resources for Biotechnology, B.E. Kirsop and C.P. Kurtzman (eds.). See Chapter 6 'Patent protection for biotechnological inventions' by I.J. Bousfield pp 141–187. Cambridge University Press, 1988.

These are written primarily for the research worker although the first two contain a considerable amount of legal and formal material of interest to the scientist who wishes to take up a career in patent law.

Advanced reading

Biotechnology and the Law, I. P. Cooper, Clark Boardman Co. Ltd, New York, 1982.
Intellectual Property Rights in Biotechnology Worldwide, S. A. Bent, R. L. Schwaab, D. G. Conlin and D. D. Jeffery, Macmillan, Stockton Press, 1987.
These books are for the patent professional reader. The authors are US attorneys but the ground covered is international, especially in Bent *et al.*

General reading and legal policy enthusiasts

Biotechnology and Patent Protection: an international review, F. K. Beier, R. S. Crespi and J. Straus, OECD, Paris, 1985.
This is a low price review available from OECD sales agents in member countries.

Index